LOSERS
KEEPERS

Lose the weight and finally keep it off for life!

Nika Ford

IMPORTANT

The information in this book reflects the authors experiences and opinions and is not intended to replace medical advice. Before beginning any nutritional or exercise regimen, consult your physician to be sure that it is appropriate for you. Readers are responsible for their own actions.

DEDICATION

This book is dedicated to all of the amazing and unique individuals who allowed me to be a part of their weight loss and weight maintenance journey. It is my heartfelt wish that you enjoy a happy, healthy, and balanced life! I am also deeply grateful to the weight loss centers I have had the privilege to work for, as well as the beautiful and sincere fellow consultants who pour their heart and souls into their client's success each and every day.

"We are each of us angels with only one wing, and we can only fly by embracing one another"

Thanks for embracing me.

Table of Contents

INTRODUCTION

MAY NOT KNOW YOU, but I will bet that you fit one of these four possibilities: You are currently on a diet, you have been on a diet in the recent past, you are contemplating beginning a new diet, or you've just finished a diet and are worried that you will gain the weight back...again.

How can I be confident that a diet is in your past, present, or future? Because more than likely you are an American citizen, and we are a nation of dieters. Statistics back me up here. The Boston Medical Center reports that approximately 45 million Americans are on a diet and that they spend about 33 billion dollars on weight loss products a year! Of course, America is not the only country getting fatter by the minute. Most so called "developed" nations are following close behind in the obesity epidemic. Yes, many countries are in a health crisis too, and people around the world are desperate to lose weight. We go on diet after diet and there are thousands of options to choose from. The majority of diets- even though they conflict and contradict each other, do work-temporarily. Here, though, is the tragic truth: it has been shown consistently that the majority of dieters will gain all of their weight back and more with each dieting attempt! You see, we know how to lose weight. We just can't figure out how to keep it off. So why do we still diet when we know that we are up against such terrible odds? Because we have hope. "This time will be different. I will be different. I will do whatever it takes to keep it off" we promise ourselves. But what does it take? Most dieters have only a vague idea, usually answering this question with something like, "Continue to be strict. Continue to eat right. Continue to exercise," but aren't all those responses really saying, "Continue to diet?"

So there is the paradox. America is on a perpetual diet and getting fatter every year. Why? Because a temporary diet will work temporarily; a perpetual diet will inevitably fail. Eventually, life will happen. We will discuss the common causes of weight regain later in this book. More importantly though, I will help you fit into that elite group of lifelong maintainers. My vision is to change the stats (and possibly the future) of those that I am privileged enough to reach and maybe even the future of the nation. Hey, it could happen!

What gives me the confidence that I can help you to achieve lifelong weight management? Because I have struggled and succeeded with maintaining a 30-pound weight loss of my own. I have learned through my own experiences, but more importantly, I have been "in the trenches" as a weight loss consultant for over 10 years. I have worked for great weight loss centers who were truly trying to help people lose weight in a healthy way. I've been blessed to work with fellow consultants who poured their heart and soul into our clients and rejoiced with them as they reached their weight loss goals. The changes that clients experienced in their lives were extraordinary: Improved energy; reduced or completely eliminated medications; a reversal of diabetes, heart disease, and many other illnesses. I've witnessed people lose from 10 lbs. to 200 lbs. I've seen self-confidence and self-respect return. Not to mention all the fun stuff- buying smaller clothes, getting compliments, wowing friends and family, or fitting into that favorite pair of jeans from 1998! I can honestly tell you that the thrill of helping people to achieve these rewards never gets old-but the heartbreak of seeing them gain it back does.

After being in the same place for years, you get to know a lot of people. The number of clients that I have been privileged to work with is in the hundreds. As consultants, we felt that we were doing our best to prepare them for maintaining their weight. We transitioned them from their weight loss menu to their maintenance menu. We encouraged them to eat healthy and offered our continued support. We implored them to check in with us on a regular basis throughout the coming year's challenges. We phoned and emailed to offer our support. More often than not, they didn't return our calls. They didn't check in and we didn't see them again until... January 1st... or the beginning of Spring... or when they outgrew everything in their closet. Or when they were diagnosed with Diabetes, high blood pressure, and so on. Here were those same clients who had shown perseverance and determination through thick and thin, who had worked so very hard to lose the weight through all manner of difficulty and who had rejoiced with us in all the blessings that weight loss bestowed upon them. Here they were returning to us with heads bowed low in shame after gaining most, if not all, of their weight back. Here they were returning in a state of final desperation to bite the bullet and do "whatever it takes" to lose the weight- again.

After years of seeing the very same clients return time and again, it really got to me. I lost joy in my work. I felt as though I was fighting a battle that could not be won. It was as if I were pulling victims out of a burning building just to watch them run back in and then cry out for help more badly burned than before. I wanted out of the weight loss world. I had had enough of the futility. I'd feel more productive banging my head against a wall! But whenever I was determined to leave, something changed my mind- the recognition that these were people-people desperately in need of help. I knew them

personally- their triumphs, their tragedies, their stories. They shared their feelings, hopes and dreams with me. They needed help. They returned time and again because they believed "this time will be different" So I felt a new passion- to make sure that it would be.

What is needed to reverse the statistics? What does it

take to be a successful weight maintainer? Two primary characteristics are required-strength and balance-physically, mentally, and emotionally. My experience with clients who have regained their weight time and again has demonstrated that having inner strength and balanced attitudes and actions were the missing link. This is no surprise in the average American's life. We burn the candle at both ends. We over eat, under sleep and drown our sorrows in food and alcohol. We feel weak emotionally and mentally, feeling the victim to circumstances. But it doesn't have to be that way. We can strengthen ourselves and create balance. Living a strong and balanced life and having a healthy relationship with food go hand in hand. Just like trying to balance on one leg, it is a skill that requires patience and practice. You may fall from time to time, but with continued practice, it becomes easier, simple, in fact.

We will take a holistic approach to weight management, one that encompasses body, mind, and spirit. By finding strength and balance not just physically, but mentally and emotionally as well, maintaining our weight is no longer a struggle but happens with ease and joy.

CHAPTER 1

CREATE A STRONG AND BALANCED BODY

Our physical experience with weight management

Food - What is it?

THE FIRST AND MOST OBVIOUS PLACE TO START would be with food. But what a perplexing issue in this day and time! What to eat has become a question with a million answers, leaving most people with a "paralysis of analysis," unable to feel confident in their choices. Advice in the area of nutrition is copious and contradictory. Foods touted as healthy abound. The phenomenon of "nutrientism," where the latest, greatest nutrient to gain popularity- Vitamin D, Omega 3's, niacin, folic acid, and such- are added to a processed food to market it as healthy. Packaging that proclaims something along the lines of "Pop Tarts, now with Omega 3's!" trick consumers into believing that junk food can magically be transformed into health food.

Michael Pollan in his book *In Defense of Food* explained that we no longer eat food, but rather, "food-like substances." He proposes a solution:

"Eat Food, not too much, mostly plants."

Simplistic, yes, but I agree wholeheartedly. People who maintain their weight for life have developed healthy taste buds. I say "developed" because for many, a taste for "plants" is an acquired one. The last two generations of Americans have largely been raised on "non- food substances." Mine was a generation of McDonalds, Taco Bell, and "home cooking" that consisted of TV dinners. The situation is worse today. The extent of many people's enjoyment of fruit and vegetables is French fries and apple pie-two for a dollar, of course!

But you were not born with the desire for processed food; That desire was learned, and it can be unlearned. The good news is that taste buds can adjust quickly, and the longer you eat real, whole, fresh, food, the more your body will crave it. Do you wonder why, if the body is supposed to crave what it needs, so many people crave unhealthy substances? This happens because our bodies are constantly working toward a state of homeostasis, one of maintaining the status quo. If we are currently in an unhealthy, toxic state, our bodies will crave what will keep us in that state. The good news is that our bodies are geniuses at adaptation. If another state-one that is clean, healthy and detoxified-is created, it will adjust to maintain that state. During your dieting phase you may have hated fruits and vegetables but ate them anyway. More than likely, you found that your taste buds changed. I can't tell you how many times a client just a few weeks into their diet exclaimed in disbelief "I actually like salads now!"

But beware. The opposite also holds true. If you begin forcing toxic, processed or "fast food" on your body it will adjust and crave those substances. Much has been written on the addictive qualities of sugar, salt and fried foods, especially when combined, as in a typical fast food meal. Renewed, repeated exposure to those foods that you gave up for your diet will inevitably overpower you and the cravings will become a fight again. So does that mean we can never eat our favorite foods again? Must we always choose foods that have optimum nutrition? Not necessarily. There is a solution. After all, no one is perfect, and there are times that we want a "not-so-clean" food, what Evelyn Tribole in *Intuitive Eating* calls "play food." Play food is food that may not have a nutritional benefit but is "fun" occasionally. I believe in balance and enjoying life. A piece of cake on your birthday, pumpkin pie on Thanksgiving, or a shared popsicle with your child on a hot summer day, these are beautiful traditions. Many people gain their weight back because they try to deny these pleasures. They have been too strict for too long and they tire out. They realize, "Hey, I want to enjoy my life!" and they believe that they must choose "fat and happy," or thin and miserable. That, fortunately, is not the case. Taste buds are very adaptive. We know that with repeated exposure to a certain food, we may "learn to like it," so too, by avoiding highly refined sugar and carbs, most find that over time their taste buds change and previously favorite foods become too sweet, too greasy or too salty. We no longer enjoy them, therefore, it is no longer a "battle" to avoid unhealthy foods. In turn, you become more sensitive to naturally sweet foods and can be very satisfied with foods such as ripe fruit for your sweet tooth. Where I used to live for candy, now a ripe, juicy peach is pure ecstasy! But occasionally you may want a not-so-virtuous "treat". The key is balance.

Balance your budget

Balancing our food intake is very much like balancing our budget. This analogy has proven the most helpful in explaining to clients how to "splurge" in moderation. I prefer the word "splurge" to "cheat." "Cheat" has shame attached. You are a free adult and can choose any food that you want. There is no "cheating." Just as you are free to spend your money any way that you want, so can you choose the food you put into your body. But if you are financially healthy, you make and follow a budget. Let's consider that. It is my guess that most of your money is spent on necessities: groceries, housing, car payments, utilities and such. But hopefully you have some left for "luxuries" or splurges. What might that be? Perhaps a new purse or shoes, or a night out to an indulgent meal or show. Occasionally you may splurge larger. Perhaps you'll go on vacation. Most likely, though, your splurges are far fewer than your spending on necessities. Your budget may change from time to time as well. If you just received a large bonus check, you may feel free to splurge a bit more. Can you see the connection? Let's explore.

Successful weight maintainers know respect their body's need for nourishment. They elevate their meals to a priority and give it necessary attention. This attention takes different forms for different people. Some just pay attention mentally, but many feel that it is very helpful to have a tracking system. I kept a food journal for several years as I learned to manage my weight. Only recently have I felt that my intuitive eating skills are strong enough that journaling is no longer necessary, but it took much time to arrive at this place of mindfulness.

Even if you eat the same thing several times a week, the act of logging my foods elevates your nutrition to a priority in my life. This is a great help if you have just come off of a diet and are learning to eat naturally again. Consider, everything important to us we "get in writing" or record in some fashion. These days' things are more commonly logged electronically, which is perfectly fine, whatever is your style. I prefer a beautiful journal and have quite a collection over the years.

By planning and tracking your food you are committing to your health. What area in your life do you have success in that you don't plan? One important common denominator with clients who regain their weight is that they eat haphazardly. With no plan, they are left wide open to be influenced by unhealthy choices. How many times have you eaten something "just because it was there?" Let's imagine instead that you had a tasty, healthy snack planned for 3 pm, and you brought it to the office with you. If a coworker brought in cookies at 2 pm, you'd be much less tempted because you had your planned, tasty snack. Yes, I said "tasty" twice. Tasty is the key. If you brought celery sticks for snack, well of course you'd want a cookie! But if you had peanut butter and a banana or a fruit and nut blend or another snack you enjoy, you could stop and reflect "My food is delicious and nutritious, I'd rather have it!"

Some people balk at the idea of planning and tracking their food. They feel that we should take a more "natural" approach to eating. I believe that at our core we are natural eaters and under perfect conditions we can trust our intuition in regard to our food choices. I strongly believe that we should honor our hunger and choose foods that are not only nutritious, but that also bring us pleasure. The reality is that we are living in a very treacherous time when it comes to eating. The book *Mindless Eating* by Brian Wansink, Ph.D, shows that numerous experiments prove that we eat or don't eat based on external cues and that paying attention to our own satiety cues is very difficult. We are influenced by our eating atmosphere, the size of the container of food, advertising, peer pressure, and much more. We are also prone to ignore signs of hunger when we feel that we are "too busy" to eat. By planning our food intake, we are overcoming outside factors. We can work intuitive eating into the picture by making sure that those foods are not only healthy but that we also enjoy them, as well as adjusting our intake based on our present hunger level. For instance, most days I feel satisfied with something such as a cup of cooked oatmeal with fruit and nuts for breakfast, so that is what I plan. If one morning for some reason I am not as hungry, I stop eating when I feel full. You are not restricted by your plan, merely guided by it. If I am still hungry, I'll eat a bit more. By all means, listen to your body and avoid a militant attitude toward eating. Planning your meals makes it easier to ensure that you take great care of yourself. You may think that you do not have time to plan your meals, but in reality, it frees up time and mental effort. You spend five minutes one time per day to plan what you will eat instead of wondering and stressing three times a day about it. As with any new undertaking, it gets easier with practice. Before long it becomes second nature. There are pros and cons to counting calories, or tracking Macronutrients-proteins, carbs, and fats. Manipulating those factors can be part of an effective diet. The challenge is to not just count and track, but listen and feel. We need to take the time to get to know ourselves and eat when we are hungry, stop when we are full, and eat food that nourishes us not just physically, but emotionally as well. There are some exceptions. If you are an athlete or body builder and are looking to build muscle or improve athletic performance, you may want to monitor your macronutrient intake. For some people however, tracking calories, fat etc. becomes an unhealthy obsession. They ignore their own hunger cues and food preferences to live strictly by the rules of the diet. You should always make sure that your eating plan has enough calories and variety to support you physically, mentally and emotionally.

Successful weight maintenance requires that you keep blood sugar stable. Drops in blood sugar result in hunger, cravings and fatigue. If you are hungry and tired you are much more likely to make a poor choice or over eat. Our brains are fueled by blood sugar. If our blood sugar drops, so does our will power. Your body overrides your best intentions and demands food. Highly refined foods raise blood sugar the quickest, so that is what we reach for. Most people feel a "crash" notoriously at 3 pm. They usually remedy the situation by grabbing a soda and candy bar or a so called "energy drink." Many others feel this drop in blood sugar in the evening between dinner and bed. A bowl of ice cream or two tends to be the only remedy. I cannot tell you of the emotional pain and embarrassment that clients feel when they relate their feelings of being weak and out of control. These are strong, successful people in other areas of their life-lawyers, CEOs, executives and so on. Think of the shame they feel when they can't stay out of the office candy bowl! They are relieved to learn of the blood sugar connection. By properly planning our meals and being diligent about eating the right foods at the right times, we greatly minimize and often eliminate hunger and cravings. That is why eating a sustaining lunch in a relaxed state is of prime importance to avoid the 3 O'clock crash. Being skillful in this area helps us regain power and control.

Get off the roller coaster!

I know firsthand the desperate and out of control feeling of being in the grips of erratic blood sugar. I was the typical teenager, running out the door to catch the bus without eating breakfast. As so many people experience, I wasn't hungry in the morning. I started feeling my hunger about 10 am. Fortunately, my school had just the solution. They sold huge pink sugar cookies and soda between classes! I remember sleeping through many of my classes, having no idea that low blood sugar was to blame. My sugar habit continued into my early adult years. I had to have sweets every day, and if I ate one, I ate three! Packages of cookies or gallons of ice cream seemed to call my name until they were gone. I remember the desperation that I felt. I gained weight rapidly after marrying at 18 years old. I gained 30 lbs in three months. I attribute this to a few things My activity level slowed down as I spent more time being a house-wife and cooking to please my new husband. I wasn't a great cook, but learned that my husband loved Velveeta, so I promptly cut off the box top and mailed it in for my first cook book- *Cooking with Velveeta*-no joke! I had quit work to be a fulltime home maker, so I had more time on my hands to eat sweets freely, and eat I did. I remember my sugar addiction being so severe that I would resolve to stop and then proudly throw the sweets in the trash. Many times when my blood sugar would plummet a couple of hours later, I returned to the trash, desperately hoping they were still on top and good enough to eat. Terrible? Yes. Uncommon? Not as much as you might think. That was the hold that sugar and out of control eating had on me. If you had told me that there would come a time when I could stop at one cookie and most often not even want one, I could not have believed it. It seemed that being the "cookie monster" was just part of who I was. And it was a part of me that I wasn't proud of. Blood sugar imbalance leads to anxiety and moodiness. Normally I was a happy, pleasant person, but not when the sugar got low! It was a "Jekyll and Hyde" effect. Learning to balance my blood sugar greatly improved not only my weight, but my quality of life and relationships- not to mention my sanity!

So how do we choose foods that best balance blood sugar? By "keeping it real." Real, whole foods provide nutrients that can be used to rebuild and repair every cell in your body. Fruits, vegetables, whole grains, and legumes are best. "If it came from the earth and it is in its whole natural form, your body can use it more effectively. The more you choose real, whole foods, the easier it will be to maintain your weight. I can guarantee you that in all my years of consulting, not once did a client ever regain their weight on fruits and veggies!

I am not against eating some process foods. After all, it's fun to have "fun food" occasionally. As with anything, balance is key. The less processed food you eat, the better your body will run and a body that is healthy and energetic is more fun than the fun-sized candy bars!

Along with choosing natural, whole foods that give your body nutrients, it is important to time those foods to keep your blood sugar stable throughout the day. Two things cause your blood sugar to drop: going too long between meals and eating highly refined sugars and starches. Let's look at the typical 3 o'clock crash. It is usually a result of an inadequate lunch or a heavy lunch, full of starchy foods. Many people skip breakfast because they don't feel hungry. But consider this, you went all night without food. Your blood sugar was already low when you woke. Your metabolism has also slowed through the night to conserve energy. You wait until noon to eat. By now you are starving, so you over eat. This rapid deluge of food, usually heavy on refined carbs, sugars and fat, causes the blood sugar to spike. What goes up, must come down, so a couple of hours later you crash.

This evil "blood sugar roller coaster" is possible to escape. It just takes diligence in the planning and preparation of your meals. Again, it doesn't have to be complicated. It just takes some forethought. Listen to your body. If you are not hungry in the morning, perhaps something small such as a piece of fruit will do. Many people are not hungry in the morning, so it is important to honor your hunger. If you are not hungry, you will likely not digest your food well. Our bodies at their natural state are in line with nature. Our digestion when regulated rises and falls like the sun. Lighter in the morning, hottest at noon and "setting" in the evening. So contrary to popular opinion, breakfast is not the most important meal of the day, lunch is. This is when our digestion works the best, properly assimilating the nutrients in our food. Remember, it's not what you eat, it's what you absorb. So if you force yourself to eat when your digestion is weak, you are not getting as much nutrition from your food.

Lunch does not get the honor it deserves in our culture. It is common for people to work through lunch. They may skip it all together, relying on caffeine to carry them through. Many others grab fast food and eat it in the car or back at their desk. Some go to a sit-down restaurant, which is an improvement over fast food, but not by much. Studies have shown that our eating environment greatly affects our food choices. Restaurant chains go to great lengths to create an environment that encourages speed and over eating. It is very difficult to be mindful of your choices and aware of your fullness in a restaurant setting. Not to mention that portion sizes are usually extreme. I am not against dining out. It can be a pleasurable experience, but for weight management, it is better to limit it to once or twice a week. Make dining out a treat, not the norm. A solution would be to pack a lunch. Again, it takes prioritizing and adjusting your routine, but think of the benefits! You are in control of your food. You know what it is and how it was prepared. You can prepare the proper portion size for yourself and not be tempted to over-eat.

Our mental state greatly affects our digestion. It has been said that "You are what you eat," but more accurately, "you are what you digest." Eating in a hurried, stressed state reduces blood flow to the stomach, causing digestion to slow. This can lead to bloating, gas, or feeling "stuffed." More importantly though, it inhibits absorption of nutrients, so even if you make a healthy choice, you are not getting the full benefit of your food. Not to be overlooked is the pleasure factor of eating. By eating slowly and mindfully, you can truly taste your food and enjoy it. By savoring your food, you will be satisfied with less. By slowing down, you may find that you really don't like the taste of your food and this can lead you to make different choices. Marc David, founder of The Institute for the Psychology of Eating, relates working with a client who wanted to lose weight but refused to stop eating his usual fast food meal for lunch. This man always went through the drive through for lunch. He ordered two large hamburgers and fries with a Coke. He was unwilling to change this habit because he believed he had to choose fast food, and he thought that he really loved his meal. Marc David took on the challenge and allowed his client to continue eating this unhealthy lunch with two stipulations: He had to park his car, instead of eating while driving. He was also instructed to truly savor his food, to eat it slowly and mindfully. What was the result? Just the act of slowing down prompted weight loss. But more importantly, he realized he really didn't like his fast food meal! The taste and the texture became very unpleasant when he was truly mindful. As a result of slowing down and being mindful, this client lost over 20 lbs. in a few short months!

I understand that sometimes our busy schedule may mean eating on the run, but that should be the exception to the rule. If this sounds familiar, ask yourself if it is necessary or just a habit. If you feel it is necessary, then work toward a more balanced schedule. Make the changes that are necessary to give your eating the attention it deserves. After all, who will take on the task of running the world, if you get sick or meet an early death due to neglecting yourself?

Now for dinner. It is a common complaint from clients that when they get home from a long, hard day's work that they are too tired to cook. So they either eat out or skip dinner and mindlessly snack all evening. I get it, I do. There are many nights that I don't get home until almost 8 pm. All I want to do is kick off my shoes and head for the couch!

Quality sleep is crucial for weight management, so if we skip dinner when we are hungry, that disrupts our sleep. If we stuff ourselves with quick, nutrient-empty convenience foods our sleep will also suffer.

What is the solution? Planning and preparation. I can hear the groans. "But I don't like to plan my meals." "I don't have time to prepare my food in advance." Well, get over it. You are reading this because you want to keep your weight off for life. If you do not take control of your life and do the work required, then get ready to be fat, sick and unhappy. Look around you. In most "developed" countries, your fellow citizens are developing heart disease, diabetes and cancer! Is that the future that you want to create? Because make no mistake, you are creating your future, one bite at a time. Every cell in your body is being repaired and renewed this very minute. This time next year, you will quite literally be a completely new person. What are you creating? Doesn't your future-self deserve to be a priority? Not to mention your present self-who you are this very minute. The food you eat causes you to feel full of life or tired and depressed. This moment is truly all we can be sure of. Did your food choices today allow you to live fully in this moment?

The good news is, it's not that hard to ensure that you have healthy meals available. It just takes some forethought. I suggest that you plan on cooking dishes that make several servings. There is no shortage of recipes for "one pot meals. Soups, chili and casseroles make great leftovers and usually taste best on the second or third day, after the flavors have had a chance to meld. One base meal can be used for a few nights without getting boring by changing the sides that you serve with it. A frequent staple in our house is beans. I will cook a pot of beans and serve them as beans and rice for the first night, then mash them and make refried beans the next night for tostados. Quickly cut some fresh tomato, onion and avocado to liven them up and your leftovers are fresh and tasty. Once you start, you will find that cooking is much easier than you think it is.

There are so many time saving options these days. Personally, I love my three tier vegetable steamer. I steam a big batch of potatoes once or twice a week to add to my meals. For breakfast, lunch, and snacks there are many no-cook options as well. Fruit and nuts, or veggies and hummus are a couple of my favorite snacks. I also occasionally use bars as a snack. But be careful here. Most so called "energy" or protein bars are, at best, glorified candy bars. The majority of them are loaded with sugar or a plethora of artificial ingredients. There are a few delicious all natural fruit and nut bars and those are my favorite when I want a convenient, sweet treat. The same goes with protein shakes. The majority are unhealthy and expensive, especially if you buy the ready-made type. But I do use some natural, plant-based protein powders that I can mix up quickly. For lunches, I love to use the packages of prewashed baby greens for my salads. Toss a few handfuls on a plate, throw some packaged sundried tomatoes, sliced almonds and pre-cooked chickpeas in the mix and voila! Gourmet salad in 30 seconds or less! Now, just try to convince me that you don't have time to eat healthy, I dare you!

I do realize that I have been doing this for a long time, and so I know the tricks and have had the practice. But if you don't start now, you will never learn the critical skill of being responsible for your own nutrition. As with any skill it takes time to "master your craft." Be patient with yourself and practice, practice, practice. You will be a pro in no time. Believe me, I got none of this growing up or during my early parenting years. Until my son was 13 years old, my idea of a well-balanced meal was Hamburger Helper, canned green beans, and white bread! But I learned, not overnight, but gradually. I changed and so can you, never doubt that. As long as you are breathing, you can learn, change, and evolve. How great is that?

Seek out the help you need if you are unsure of yourself in the kitchen. Information abounds on creating quick, easy and tasty meals. In our information age, there is no excuse for not learning what you need to know. It just takes the courage to face the challenge and the humility to ask for help. Don't be embarrassed. Cooking has become an almost lost art, especially preparing healthy meals. But there are few skills more important to your health, wellbeing, and weight management. So "just do it," okay? The time and effort invested will pay off in the quality and perhaps quantity of life!

Exercise-Is it necessary?

We covered eating right, now we will cover exercise. After all, if there is a universal answer to how to lose weight and keep it off, it would be to "eat right and exercise," and, in a nutshell, that is technically correct.

But we are not "nuts," (Most of us aren't, anyway!) We are amazingly complex beings, so the answer is much more complex. Of course, exercise is an undeniable component of weight management, so we will address this as the second aspect of creating a balanced body.

Look at your body-literally. Pause for a moment and really look at your body. Look beyond the skin and underlying fat and suspend judgment for a moment. Now look with your mind's eye to a deeper level, to your muscles. Visualize your body as an anatomy chart. You know the one with the red man illustrating all of his muscles? That's you, underneath it all. There are approximately 650 muscles in your body- yes, yours. They may not be developed in a way that makes them obvious, but they are there. Why? Because we are made to move! And once upon a time we did. Visualize the hunter/gatherer in a running stride, arm outstretched, brandishing a spear; or the pioneer clearing the land, building the house, cultivating the ground; or the housewife a few generations ago, scrubbing the clothes on the washboard and then carrying her heavy basket to hang them out to dry. Wow, how times have changed, and thank goodness they have! Believe me, I am a great fan of progress and convenience and am not here advocating a "return to nature" approach to living in this regard. I love my dishwasher as much as the next girl, but I think you see my point. There was a time that the admonition to "get some exercise" was virtually unheard of.

The situation is very different today. Many Americans lead sedentary lives. Approximately 28 % are completely sedentary, and 192 million Americans are not active to healthy standards. Advances in technology make it increasingly rare to have to expend significant physical effort in our day to day lives. The evidence proves that if you expect to maintain a healthy weight for life, you will need an active lifestyle. Some people are naturally active and have no need to schedule formal exercise into their day. My friend Shelly has maintained her 20 lb weight loss for over three years. When I asked her what type of exercise she does, she gave me a slightly guilty grin and said, "I don't!" If you met Shelly, you would understand; she is the human equivalent of the "Energizer Bunny!" She lives on fast forward. It is torture for her to sit still. She is also a very involved mom to her 8-year-old daughter Kayla. Their time is spent riding bikes, gardening, swimming, having water balloon fights, you name it. Shelly is the polar opposite of sedentary. But she is the exception to the rule. So unless your friends would describe you as the "Energizer Bunny" you're probably going to have to exercise like the rest of us!

Exercise is not a chore; it is a gift. Yes, I can see some rolling their eyes at me, like I'm Mom telling little Johnnie that eating his spinach will make him strong like Popeye, but it is true. Feeling your muscles, lungs, and heart working and seeing them improve over time is a true thrill. The secret is in how you approach exercise. If it is a "necessary evil" to keep from gaining weight, of course you will avoid it. But if you find activities that you enjoy, do well, and can see continued progress, then you will look forward to it.

The National Weight Control Registry tracks those who have lost 30 lbs. or more and have maintained for over a year. They found that the preferred exercise among maintainers was walking. The average was one hour of walking, five days a week. So if you enjoy walking, walk a lot. The key to success is consistency. But just because walking is the most common exercise doesn't mean it's the best for you. The key is choosing what is best for you as an individual.

Do what you love

What physical activities do you enjoy? What makes you feel strong, energetic, and happy? The possibilities are endless! Walking, running, dancing, skating, karate, boxing, Zumba, swimming, water aerobics, belly dancing, hiking, kick boxing, Pilates, yoga, hula hooping, skiing, rock climbing, shall I go on?

My goal for exercise keeps with the premise of this book-strength and balance. My two current favorite activities are strength training with weights and yoga. First, let's look at weight training. Yes, I love to "pump the iron." Why? Because feeling my strength and sculpting my body benefit me not just physically, but mentally and emotionally, in a way that nothing else does. I haven't always felt this way. I remember a time as a young adult when a friend squeezed my soft, small arm where a bicep was nonexistent and called me "weak as a cat." I laughed at him in surprise and exclaimed, "What? Do you want me to be a *man*?" Muscles were of no interest to me. As many women fear, I felt that muscle would make me "manly." But my viewpoint changed as I got older. I came to see that women as well as men needed strength and that a gaining muscle was a good thing.

Growing up, I had no athletic or competitive nature at all. I was always last pick for the team in P.E. I was never involved or remotely interested in sports. I stayed active by walking around the neighborhood or typical kid activities like roller skating and riding my bike. The concept of training for strength was new to me. I lifted my first dumbbell at about age 30, and saw some progress in my efforts to strengthen and tone my body, but I was very sporadic in my efforts. I had enough of a taste of strength, though, that I knew what weight bearing exercise could do for me; it could lead to not only physical strength, but psychological strength as well. This is what Bill Phillips in his book *Body for Life* refers to as the "power mind-set."

In 2005 I left a very dysfunctional marriage of 16 years and set out to build a new life for myself and pre-teen son. I left with just the possessions I could fit in my car. I was on my own for the first time since I was eighteen years old. Here I was, a 35 years old, single mom working two jobs. (My second job was as a waitress at Denny's and many nights I didn't get home until 2 am.) My need for the "power mind-set" was more than my need to breathe! I joined a 12-week challenge and lost 20 lbs. What's more, I learned the crucial truth that we are stronger than we know. It is no exaggeration to say that strength training was a key factor in my surviving a terribly difficult divorce and turning my life from negative to positive, as well as being a physical cornerstone to all of the success that I have experienced in the last 10 years.

Another set of circumstances calling for mental and physical strength happened in January of 2011 when I helped my mom escape a life-threatening, abusive relationship. Not many months later she was diagnosed with inoperable cancer and I became her sole caregiver for 15 months. Throughout this time, I renewed my commitment to strength training. I knew that by becoming stronger physically, I would be stronger mentally and emotionally to be the support that she needed. I was able to "hold it together" and be strong for her until her passing. I practiced yoga and meditation as well, giving me the "balance" part of the equation. Yoga gave me a different strength of spirit and a calm centeredness as well. This combined aspect of physical, mental, and emotional strength and balance enabled me to help make Mom's last days some of our best ones together.

My reason for including a mini-autobiography of the last 13 years of my life is this: to help you to appreciate the power of exercise. Weight training or yoga may not be your thing, but feeling your physical strength and power in some way can be the foundation for taking control of your life, as well as your weight.

Progress-The key to happiness

Tony Robbins, in his life-changing motivational seminars, frequently stresses that to be truly happy in life we need to see ourselves making progress. Much of why a person is successful on a diet is the thrill of seeing their own progress. They see the number on the scale go down, inch loss increase, and their clothes getting looser. They hear praise from family and friends. When the weight loss is over, that thrill of progress is gone as well. Many then find themselves in a state of wandering aimlessly in the desert of everyday life. This "what next?" stage can be discouraging. The key is to set goals that allow you to see constant improvement. Fitness goals not only keep your body healthy but give your mind and spirit the thrill and sense of accomplishment they crave.

What might our fitness goals be? Again, weight training is perfect for seeing our own progress and improvement. We can set goals to lift heavier or do more repetitions. We can track our progress each work out for instant feedback. Consider this amazing marvel of the human body: it will adapt to meet the demand placed upon it. Muscles grow as a result of a physical demand placed upon them that they are challenged to meet. When we lift heavy enough to put demand on our muscle, it creates tiny microscopic tears in the muscle. This is why, if you pushed yourself in the gym today, tomorrow you will most likely experience what is referred to as DOMS- delayed onset muscle soreness. This could mean that you have difficulty walking for the next day or two! When your muscles are strained in this way, the body goes to work repairing those tiny tears by laying down new muscle fiber. This layering effect creates more muscle, thereby causing your muscles to grow. With time and consistency, this allows you to lift increasingly heavier weight. How amazing is that? It's like the body says "Hey, that was hard! I need to get better prepared for the next time!"

I am in awe of the human body and its capabilities. The thrill of seeing an increase in our own strength is something that I wish more people would experience. When you start out lifting five pound dumbbells, and then one day you are doing the same exercise with 20 pounds, you feel pretty tough!

Many women are uncomfortable in the gym. They feel intimidated by the other women that are fitter than they are. But remember that everyone had to start somewhere. And then there are the guys! Don't be intimidated by the men in the gym. They usually lift heavy so you may hear some grunting or slamming of weights depending on your gym. But don't worry about them watching you. In most cases they are too busy looking at themselves in the mirror! If you can't get over your insecurity in the gym, you can work out at home or join a "women only" gym. Personally, "women only" gyms make me cringe. How can we voluntarily segregate ourselves? Women have fought long and hard to be equal to men. The first female marathon runner was beaten by a mob for taking part in a "man's race." I empathize if you feel insecure in the gym, but I strongly urge you to get over it. You are a strong, capable woman. All you need is knowledge and experience to feel right at home in a gym setting. Most gyms offer a complimentary training session to show you how the machines work. So put your big girl panties on and do it! You will begin to live for the thrill of feeling your strength and endurance increase. Oh yeah, did I mention that seeing your body become tight and sculpted is pretty great too? Exercise can give you an ongoing sense of accomplishment, and think of how much more fun it is to "eat right and exercise" to get stronger, instead of just smaller.

Any activity done purposefully and mindfully can provide you with a sense of progress and accomplishment. A popular program for running called "Couch to 5K" allows would-be runners to set incremental goals to improve their running in preparation for entering a 5K race. If you are one who prefers to "do your own thing" as I do, then progress could be made by reaching goals such as decreasing your minutes per mile or increasing the distance you run. When your 1-mile run used to take 30 minutes and now it takes 15, that's exciting! If you would rather just walk, that is fine, but be purposeful and set goals to measure your progress. Increase your speed or duration. Add some inclines. Consistently reaching your goals brings an excitement to life. Henry Ford said "Enthusiasm is at the bottom of all progress" in turn, I say, "Progress is the basis for enthusiasm." Fuel your fire with progressive exercise goals.

What are some other examples of activities that keep you fit and fuel your "zest for life?" Perhaps you would like to learn to dance. The possibilities are endless! Ballroom, swing, hip hop, jazz and the very popular dance-fitness craze, Zumba. I have recently begun

Zumba, and I am already a huge fan! It is the perfect "lighter side" to my weight-training and yoga. The only skill needed is the ability to laugh at yourself and have fun! I love to see all shapes and sizes dancing and enjoying themselves. I see it as a great activity to build a healthy body image. The classes I've attended were vocal, filled with "whoops and hollers" as well as laughter. Laughter in itself lowers cortisol production, helping to burn belly fat. Classes abound, but you can also practice at home through video. Progress is felt when you learn the moves and are able to become more skilled in the routine with less effort.

Yoga is another great activity to gauge your progress. Don't be intimidated by yoga. It is not about becoming a human pretzel. Actually, that is never necessary. Yoga simply means "union" or "yoking." It is a union of the breath with the body, the body with the mind and spirit. There are as many styles of yoga as there are of dance, so find one that fits your personality and needs. Gentle or restorative, hot yoga or flow yoga, Yin or Yang, there is something for everyone. Yoga can be spiritual or not. If you are only interested in yoga to increase flexibility and strength, yoga classes taught at a gym are usually purely physical. If you are interested in exploring the spiritual benefits of yoga, look for a studio. Read the descriptions. *The Complete Idiots Guide to Yoga* is a great aid for understanding the history as well as current styles of yoga. No matter which style you choose, you will experience a greater connection to your body. Yoga links breath to body. This becomes a "meditation in motion," calming the restless mind. You can feel your muscles work in a way they may never have before. Many find that their self-esteem and body confidence greatly improve when they practice yoga. If your body type doesn't fit the yoga image of a young, thin, white girl, know that this image is completely fabricated by the media. Yoga is for everyone. Pick up an authentic Yoga manual and you're likely to see a dark skinned, hairy and not-too-buff, middle-aged man! Yoga teaches you to respect your true self and to connect with your body. Anyone can see progress and progress equals happiness. The day you can hold "tree pose" without wobbling, you will know what I mean!

I have begun to incorporate variety into my exercise regimen and am loving the multitude of benefits, physically, mentally and emotionally. Weight training makes me feel like a bad-ass. Yoga makes me feel enlightened, and Zumba reminds me I'm a dork and need to lighten up and have fun!

We have discussed several options for exercise. Many times I hear people say that they can't exercise because of certain physical limitations. You may have some very legitimate limits. Maybe you have a disease or disorder that makes certain exercises painful or impossible. I truly empathize with you. But I also hope to inspire you to ask "What can I do?" If any part of your body moves, move it! Yes, your progress will be slower than someone with no health issues. Acknowledge that. But think of the people you will inspire. You will be able to say "I did it even though I have this (disease, disorder, difficulty) and so can you!"

My friend Joyce is a great example of this. She is in her 60's. A couple of years ago she had heart trouble and had to have a pacemaker put in. Strenuous exercise is out of the question. But Joyce doesn't let that keep her from being active every day. Joyce walks. She's not speedy, but she's consistent. She has a fabulous way to stay motivated and see progress. Joyce determines how many miles she wants to walk in a year. Last year she walked 400! When I saw her this September, she told me that she was on track to reach 500 miles by the end of this year. The ear-to-ear grin on her face as she told me she could've walked "halfway to Colorado" shows how exciting it is to set exercise goals and reach them. Joyce is a great example of following the admonition to "do what you can, with what you have, where you are."

It is not my purpose to give you a workout routine to follow, just as I didn't give you specific meal plans. I am here to motivate you to take action to find healthy food and physical activity that fits you. What works for me isn't necessarily best for you. Take the time to find your fit. Resources abound. There is no shortage of recipes and exercise routines in print or online. Be intuitive, listen to your body, and choose food and activity that makes you feel alive. Then weight management is an exciting adventure, not a necessary evil.

KEYS TO CREATING A STRONG AND BALANCED BODY

Make healthy eating a priority

Get in touch with your true hunger and take the time to prepare nourishing foods

Eat tasty food that you enjoy

Be active on most days of the week

Choose enjoyable, yet challenging, exercise that allows you to see progress

CHAPTER 2
CREATE A STRONG AND BALANCED MIND

Getting our brain on board

S O WE HAVE COVERED "EAT RIGHT AND EXERCISE." What more could there be to discuss? After all, isn't that all you need to do to maintain a healthy weight? Well, if we were little equations of calories in and calories out, it would be. And up until pretty recently, that was the mantra chanted in most weight loss circles. But ever increasing light is being shed on the mind-body connection. It is a well-established fact that our mind can cause or cure disease. We know of the "placebo effect" where just believing that an inactive substance is strong medicine causes the patient to get well. It is also widely accepted that a patient with a life-threatening disease who has hope and a positive disposition is much more likely to recover; whereas a patient who is depressed and believes that he will die is much more likely to. Most people would also agree that being in a stressed state can cause a heart attack. Think of that. Our mindset and "inner voice" can cause or cure disease! Why wouldn't it also cause or prevent weight gain? So our mental state is important to our health. Our thoughts actually change our body chemistry. Stressful feelings cause an imbalance of the hormone Cortisol. Cortisol imbalance leads to belly fat. So our mind and the thoughts we think directly influence hormone production, making it harder to lose weight and keep it off.

Silence the voices in your head

Another simple fact that illustrates how our mind affects our body is that we "do what the voices in our head tell us to." Our inner dialog can be our best friend or our worst enemy. The things that many people say to themselves are heart breaking. "I have no will power" "I deserve to be fat" I'll never keep this weight off." "Who am I fooling?" "I shouldn't have eaten that" "I'm bad" "I cheated" "I'm so stupid!" "I can't have that." "I can't stop with just one." "I have no control." On and on the mental beatings continue, hour after hour, day after day. And just as with getting physically tortured long enough and hard enough, we are bound to break. We become what we think. Buddha said it best-

"All that we are is the result of what we have thought. With our thoughts we create our world."

So if you envision your world as a happy, healthy one

where you will never need to diet again, then you must learn to control the voices in your head.

Many of us who have dieted frequently have developed what I call the "diet martyr" mentality. That is a mind full of rules, "shoulds" and "shouldn'ts" and the accompanying guilt resulting from breaking those rules. Our minds are full of "the good, the bad and the ugly"- judgments of our food and our choices. Most of the time, we don't even realize what has led us to label certain foods as good or bad. Was it a forbidden food on a previous diet? Was it a study touting the dangers or benefits of a certain food? Did Mom tell you that you "shouldn't eat that?" We usually don't question the rules that we have picked up along the way, but we allow the breaking of those rules to cause us guilt and shame. Guilt and shame are not productive, especially when there is no sound basis for them. Linda Spangle, author of *Life is Hard, Food is Easy* emphasizes that guilt has no place in our food choices. She discusses the common expression that we "cheated" by eating a certain food. Cheating is committing an act that is illegal or immoral. Food is neither one. Did you steal the food? Did you kill someone for it? No? Then no need to feel guilty.

You are free to choose

Our food choices are just that-choices. Some are more nutritious than others. Some will support your health and weight maintenance goals, some will not. But they are not good, bad, right or wrong. You may set standards for yourself as to what you will and will not eat and, by all means, I do encourage you to have standards! I do my best to avoid foods that I know are damaging to my health or to my wellbeing. This means that I avoid foods that are empty nutritionally and contain artificial toxins. I also avoid foods that trouble my spirit because they were produced through suffering, such as meat and factory farmed dairy. This is the standard that I have chosen. The key is "I" and "choose." At any time, I know that I can choose differently. If one day I decide that I want a Twinkie with a glass a milk, that is my choice. (My friends and family would suspect alien abduction if they saw me eating a Twinkie, but nevertheless, it's my choice.)

We humans inevitably desire the "forbidden fruit." If we are told no, we are naturally inclined to want what we can't have. By labeling a food as bad or telling ourselves "I can't have chocolate," we set ourselves up for failure. How many times have you eaten the whole gallon of ice cream or package of cookies just to "get it out of the house, because I 'm never buying it again?" But if you know that you can have it anytime, it loses its "Last Meal" importance.

"Take away the object of my desire, and I will fight you for it. Take away my desire for the object, and I willingly surrender it."

How much more empowering is it to tell ourselves, "I choose to avoid sugar because I want to create a healthy body" or "I choose to avoid fast food because I want to nourish my body with real food?" At any time, we have the power to choose differently. My friends and family know that I eat healthy most of the time, but occasionally they will offer me something with the question, "Can you have that?" I can't help but emphatically answer, "I can have anything I want! I *choose* not to." As a weight loss coach, I am constantly asked by clients "Can I have ...on this program?" My answer is always, "You can have anything you want, but for best results, I recommend this." Would they rather have a simple yes or no answer? Of course. So many people say "Just tell me what to do!" But who am I to tell you what you can or can't do? You are a free adult. I can give you guidance, but you get to choose. How great is that?

Don't underestimate the importance of this. I have seen so many people stick to a strict diet for months without compromise only to "spontaneously combust" and go crazy, eating anything and everything until they gain all of their weight back. I have many times seen clients lose 100 lbs. or more. Think of that. For approximately a full year, they were strict through trials and tribulation. They prided themselves on their will power and the accompanying success they experienced. But almost inevitably they gained it back with a vengeance. Why? Because they had been restricted the longest. This is one prime factor, but other factors come into play, such as lacking the humility to ask for help. We will discuss that more later.

We can only say no to ourselves for so long. We are made to be rebels, to crave freedom, to fight restrictions. Look at the Prohibition, did it prevent alcohol consumption? No. People became willing to risk jail and even death to get what they were denied. I do not believe in black and white rules and restrictions, rather, I believe in education and freedom of choice as to whether you will act on that knowledge. We will discuss more on the education part, but please rid yourself of "can't," "shouldn't," "bad," "cheat," etc. Claim your freedom and use it responsibly!

"You're not dead. Learn."

Those words were bluntly spoken to me by a stranger when I was 29 years old. I was working in the coffee shop of Books-a-Million at the time. I don't remember the actual conversation, only that it involved geography and somehow I was forced to expose the fact that I am embarrassingly ignorant on the subject. I couldn't tell you if Africa is closer to South America or Europe. I could probably identify only about half of the states on a U.S. map. I know, I told you it was embarrassing. My excuse is this-I was not interested in geography in school, or as a matter of fact, anything really, except drama and creative writing. Yep, I'm the poster child for "right brained." My mother was great, but pretty much uninvolved in my academic endeavors. There was no one in my life that helped me see the importance of studying the boring subjects like history, math and geography. And I saw no need, since I was *sure* to be a famous writer and actress, with no need for such useless knowledge!

Most of the time I can avoid revealing my lack of left-braininess. I know enough math to get me by. But when geography or history surfaces, I politely exit the conversation. On occasion when my ignorance is exposed, I laugh my way out of it with a cute little, "I slept through that class" or "I only studied boys" or the repentant, "I wish I would've paid more attention in school." Most people would just nod politely and kindly excuse my ignorance. Not this lady! When I offered the repentant excuse, she looked me in the eye very unsympathetically and with cold, harsh clarity replied "You work in a bookstore. You're not dead. Learn!" Well, that hit home. While it did not compel me to learn geography, because truthfully, it's just not a priority, it did pull the rug out from under 11 years of excuses. Yes, I am no longer in school, but I am still breathing. No longer will I allow myself to be satisfied with "I don't know" or "I never learned that" because I have faced the truth that ignorance is willful, and that, if I really want to, I can choose to learn anything.

Nutrition is probably not something that you learned in school. Even doctors rarely get more than a few hours' worth of nutritional education. I spoke with a head nurse who was confused as to why her tator tots were not a weight-loss choice since they were "organic!" My clients are mostly highly educated professionals with degrees-doctors, nurses, teachers, executives. When they must admit that they don't know if oatmeal is a protein or a carb, it's embarrassing to them. But as with history and geography, or even reading and writing, for that matter, we are not born with it, but we can learn.

Where do we start? That's a tough question. As I was encouraging a client to reflect on her choices and if they benefited her health, I suggested she ask herself as she ate the Milk Duds that she thought she couldn't resist-"What great thing is this doing for my body?" and to choose food that nourished her with lots of nutrients. When she asked in frustration "But how do I *know* which foods are good for me?" It was a real eye opener to me. While it was obvious to me that a box of Milk Duds only hurt her health, it was a revelation to her. Just as with the organic tator tots, many people are clueless about healthy choices.

It reminded me that I am much further "down the path" regarding nutritional knowledge. It's always humbling for me to remember the clueless, sugar-addicted version of me in my early 20's. Do you remember the "fat-free" craze of the 1990's? I do. I had gained weight rapidly after marrying at 18 yrs old. I had never dieted before then. So when I found myself 30lbs overweight I tried to figure out what to do. "Stop eating crap" never occurred to me. So, like most, I searched for the weight loss "secret" that would allow me to eat all the sweets I wanted and lose weight. Here was the miracle that would let me do that- just choose "fat free!" That made perfect sense, eating fat made you fat, well of course! How exciting! All I had to do was look for fat free candy, and guess what? There is a lot. My favorite was candy corn. I could buy two bags for a buck, and I did, frequently. I can still remember my older, wiser friend questioning me about my two-bag-a-day habit. I also remember my confusion at her eye roll when I exclaimed, "What? They're fat free!" Kind of sounds like tator tot lady, doesn't it?

Yes, I have come a long way, baby. And so can you. Now, if you lost weight by choosing whole foods, such as fruits, vegetables and lean proteins, then you are off to a great start to choosing foods that will help you maintain. But if your diets have been those that consisted of pre-packaged meals or meal replacement shakes or diet pills or a miracle cleanse, etc. then you may have never really learned nutrition. It is difficult to retrace the steps that brought me to where I am nutritionally, and I want to shorten the process for you. So where to start? I suggest that before you begin scrutinizing labels and reading books on nutrition that you step back and get in touch with something we all possess, but often don't trust: Common Sense.

Educated Eating

There is a crisis in this country. An epidemic of immense proportions. This epidemic affects our very brain. It specifically targets the area of our brain that is responsible for our inherent knowledge, our so called "common sense." This epidemic is called "paralysis of analysis." There was a time when people knew what food was. It was obvious. Food grew from the ground, or was made from plants that grew from the ground. They grew it or picked it or bought it from someone they knew. This food did not come with labels. There was no turning the orange over to check the nutrient facts to see how many carbs it contained. If it was ripe, you picked it, you ate it, and you loved it! Of course you did, because it was sweet and juicy, blessed by the sun and rain and full of nutrients from the rich soil. You didn't need a label to tell you that you should eat it for the fiber or vitamin C. You knew intuitively that you should eat it. The enticing scent and vibrant color attracted you, and you felt refreshed and nourished by eating it.

The situation is so much more complicated today. We have all but lost our "natural" ability to choose food. Most people in the developed nations have trouble even discerning what real food is. We are tricked by artificial colors and flavors to make products that are unnatural seem appealing. Then we are bombarded with so called nutrient facts to cast a halo or devil horns on a particular product. For these reasons and much more, we are "paralyzed" when it comes to choosing our foods.

Instead of trusting our senses we are influenced by advertising or the latest so called "scientific" study about the latest super nutrient. I would like to make it so much more simple for you. Choose the vast majority of your foods from the "no labels." Create your meals and snacks primarily from fruits vegetables, nuts, seeds and whole grains, (the actual grain, like oats and rice and not "whole grain" processed products). I guarantee you that I have never seen anyone regain their weight from eating real, whole foods. It does not happen!

I am not opposed to eating some minimally processed food. Natural peanut butter (containing only peanuts and salt) is a daily staple for me. I also drink store bought almond milk, because, quite frankly, I don't want the hassle of making my own. I like a fruit and nut bar or high-quality protein bar as an occasional treat. I don't think it is necessary or realistic to never eat packaged food, but if you make them the exception to the rule, you will find maintaining your weight almost a given.

In my experience, people regain their weight almost invariably through processed, refined products, what Micheal Pollan calls "food-like substances." So many times we get caught up in choosing a food based on what it is not. It's not high in fat, or carbs or calories. Many clients feel virtuous when they mention to me that they chose a 100 calorie "snack pack" for their snack. I recently had a client bring one of those in to ask what I thought of it. "It's only 100 calories," she said, proudly. I flipped the wrapper over and showed her the ingredient list and asked her "100 calories of *what*?" She scanned the paragraph-long list of unpronounceable ingredients and looked bewildered. "What great nutrition is this giving your body?" I asked. "Nothing," she conceded. I then went on to give her quick and easy real food snack options.

There is a natural progression that happens when we begin to become aware of our food choices that I have experienced myself and have witnessed in others. This usually begins with our first diet. We begin to read labels, starting with that handy, dandy little box:

"Nutrient Facts." First, we look at the calories in the food and aim to choose items with the least calories. As we evolve as savvy dieters, we begin to look at the fat and carb grams. We may even begin to notice the grams of sugar or salt. We know that being "good" means choosing foods that are low in all of these. As our health IQ improves, we start looking for things that our foods are "high" in: high protein, high fiber, high monounsaturated fat and so on. We learn to examine and evaluate the "facts" of our food. But rarely do we ask ourselves "What is it?" I know in my case I was many years deep into my weight loss career, before I asked myself that question. The epiphany hit me over a bowl of fat-free, sugar-free Cool Whip. I loved the stuff! I would pile it high on my hot chocolate or my sugar-free Jell-O. I would crown a beautiful bowl of strawberries with it. When mixed with peanut butter, it was to die for! I never even felt a tinge of guilt when I ate it straight from the container. After all, it was "free," 10 calories, no fat, no sugar. It was a puffy white cloud of virtuous, heavenly bliss. But for some reason, one day as I indulged freely, I looked, not at the saintly nutrition facts, but at the ingredients.

Ingredients

Water, Corn Syrup, High Fructose Corn Syrup, Vegetable(s) Oil Hydrogenated (Coconut Oil, Palm Kernel Oil), Sodium Caseinate from milk, Flavor(s) Natural & Artificial, Corn Starch Modified, Xanthan Gum, Guar

Gum, Polysorbate 60, Sorbitan Monostearate, Sodium Polyphosphate, Acesulfate

What the @#$%?!

It was then that it hit me. I almost threw the bowl across the room in disgust. I also shook my head at my own ignorance and the fact that I was a health educator and had still, after all this time, been duped by its innocent appearance. I have since begun to refer to it by a more accurate name: "Chemical Whip." Still, when compared to many foods, that is a very short list of ingredients!

My Chemical Whip revelation is when I began to actually ask, "What *is* it?" This obvious question is not so obvious to most of us. Most of us have grown up in the age of packaged foods and serpentine marketing. It takes extraordinary sense to use common sense.

If you looked at the above ingredients and responded with "so what?" then I encourage you to do some research. Look up those ingredients. You would have to live under a rock to have not heard of the dangers of high fructose corn syrup, as well as the dangers of chemicals and artificial ingredients in our food. So if you are just now emerging from your rock, do yourself a favor and start to Google your ingredients before you guzzle them! Remember, our very lives are dependent on the food that we ingest. Isn't it worth some time to find out what materials you are building your future self with? You may have never really been aware of the dangers in our food supply, but remember, "You're not dead. Learn."

You can amass a huge file on the dangers of chemicals and artificial ingredients in our food to defend your reasons to avoid them, or you can use the short answer that I prefer: "Because they are artificial." Duh.

But what does artificial mean, anyway?

ar·ti·fi·cial

adjective \ˌär-tə-ˈfi-shəl\

: not natural or real: made, produced, or done to seem like something natural

: not happening or existing naturally: created or caused by people

: not sincere

Not natural. Not real. Created by people. That pretty much sums it up.

I truly believe that we come from the earth and are part of the earth. We are designed to be nourished by the earth. When we eat foods that come from the earth, our bodies recognize and assimilate them, drawing nutrients and nourishment from them. Our body has a purpose for the ingredients found in nature, a "home" for them. The way that we are sustained through food is truly an incomprehensible miracle. But when these artificial ingredients enter into our systems, our bodies don't know what to do with them. There is no purpose for "polysorbate 60" in our genes. Therefore, our bodies must find a place for them. These toxins are stored in our fat cells. Our bodies must create more fat cells to have a place for them.

To illustrate this, think about all those little irritating items lying around your house that you don't have a use for. You don't throw them away, because you think that you might need them someday. I would bet that you have what is known as a "junk drawer," a catch-all for the crap that you don't know what to do with. The more junk you have; the more space you need to store it. First it's a drawer, then a closet, then perhaps you have a junk room to store all of it. Sometimes the junk fills a whole house, as the terrible TV shows on "hoarders" make us painfully aware. Well, think of artificial ingredients as junk, and your fat cells as drawers. It is not obvious to our body that these ingredients should be thrown away. After all, the definition of artificial also said "something done to seem like something real" All of this stored artificial junk can overwhelm our bodies and damage not only our waistline, but also our overall health.

Do you know how good it feels to live in a clean, uncluttered home? If you have lived in a disorganized, messy environment for a long time, it can be very difficult to feel motivated to clean it up. But once you do, you most likely will feel that it is worth the effort to keep it clean. It is the same with our food choices. Getting rid of the "junk" in our diet can be overwhelming at first. The key is to take it one "room" at a time. Don't expect to change everything at once.

Small steps on a consistent basis lead to big changes. The first step is awareness. Begin by asking the magic question "What is it?" and strive to primarily choose foods that you can confidently say are real and not made to "seem that they are real." In time, living in a clean body will make you wonder how you could ever have "trashed" it in the first place!

Mindful Eating

We have also not learned to trust our common sense when it comes to the *amount* of food that we eat. Many of us have never known what it is like to eat "naturally." Many women had mothers who were chronic dieters, so they were raised from a young age with the example of counting calories or fat grams or drinking diet shakes or eating "lean" frozen dinners. The idea of listening to your hunger level and choosing whole, real foods is a new thought for many. I can tell you that until pretty recently, I felt that it was necessary to track, if not calories, than at least protein and carbs to make sure I got the right balance. I wouldn't eat peanut butter unless I pulled out the tablespoon or oatmeal without the measuring cup. The idea of saying "How much do I want?" instead of "What's the proper serving size?" was scary. It was difficult for me to put the measuring cups away and ask myself "What is a reasonable amount of this food? What will make me feel satisfied without being too much?" I had to trust that I knew what was best for me, but over time I have become more secure in my food intuition. As I discussed earlier though, "intuitive eating" is difficult because we are influenced so much by outside factors. I also don't believe in "flying by the seat of our pants" regarding our meal choices. I believe we need to plan and prepare our food ahead of time if we want to be successful at managing our weight. We generally know what it will take to feel satisfied. If we pack our lunch, we can usually guess how much it will take to satisfy us. If at lunch time we get full before we are finished, we can stop eating instead of saying, "I need exactly 4 oz. of protein so I will make myself eat this." That type of rigidity has proven helpful for weight loss, where the right ratios of protein to carbs and calorie counting are helpful, but it is not necessary for maintenance.

Most likely you lost your weight on a diet that predetermined what the right amount of food was for you, instead of relying on your natural intuition. That is because burning fat is unnatural. We are much more disposed to store fat. It's a basic and marvelous survival mechanism. So losing weight quickly, requires manipulating our bodies in an unnatural way. During dieting you were likely taught to ignore your hunger and to eat, even though you were full, or to stop eating, even though you were still hungry when your prescribed amount was gone. This may have enabled you to lose weight, but it is counterintuitive for lifelong weight management. I believe that this militant attitude to food can actually sabotage your weight maintenance efforts.

Why? Simply because it is impersonal and unreliable.

Our bodies are not all the same. You never really know how many calories, protein, carbs and fat grams you truly need. One day differs from the next. I can tell you that on days that I wake up at early and weight train heavily, I'm hungry! I need more food than on days that I wake up later and go for a light walk. When I'm about to start my period I am hungrier than other times of the month. So I eat more at those times. This is the "common sense" I was talking about. If my goal was, for instance, 1500 calories a day, I'm going to be too full some days and too weak and hungry on the others.

Then there is our rebel nature. If I strictly adhere to 1500 calories daily, eventually I will get sick and tired of being so damn perfect all the time, and dive into the deep end of "fat and happy" land. This hedonism will last until my emerging muffin top forces me to once again chain myself to my calorie counter. Enough already! Calorie tracking has proven very helpful to many dieters, but I believe it is unnecessary and possibly counterproductive to life-long weight management.

It can be frightening to learn to trust yourself and your body. It is a process and a skill that takes time. Be patient with yourself. Learn to honor your hunger, choose real food, and eat mindfully. In this way you will maintain your weight-and your sanity.

The way to eat

So what does it mean to eat "mindfully?" Well, simply

put, it means that when you eat, eat. Don't watch TV, check email, drive, talk on the phone or a hundred different activities that we think we must do. This ridiculous multitasking that we pride ourselves on sabotages our weight in at least three ways. First, as I described earlier with the client of Marc David who ate lunch in his car every day, the act of eating on the run stresses your body. When our body is under stress it does not assimilate nutrients well. So even if you are eating the purest organic foodstuffs on the planet, you are not getting the full benefit if you are watching the nightly news report of doom and gloom. Secondly, mindless eating prevents you from noticing when you are full. Have you ever had the experience of reaching into the bag of chips and finding that they are all gone and asking "How did that happen?" It happened because your hand was in contact with your mouth but not your brain! The third, and I feel the most important, harm in mindless eating is that you don't get the full enjoyment of your food; many times you aren't even tasting it. We are left yearning for more and are never truly satisfied. When we take the time to savor our food, we find that we are much happier with a little of the good stuff than a whole lot of the junk. Let's consider two different scenarios to illustrate the point.

First scenario: You are on your lunch break. You want chocolate. You whip into the corner convenience store and are happy to discover that the candy bars are on sale- two for the price of one! "Sweet!" They're not your favorite, but hey, they're a bargain. You only wanted one, but couldn't pass up the deal. You assure yourself that you will save one or maybe give it to your coworker Sue, because you're thoughtful like that. On your way to the car, you open one candy bar and take a bite. As you drive back to work, you finish the bar in several large bites as you tune the radio, curse the driver who cut you off and watch the clock, worried you'd get back to work late. "Damn this Friday traffic! Hey, what happened to my candy bar? Gone already? Thank God I bought two. With all this stress I could use another one! Sue doesn't know I was planning on giving it to her anyway; Oh, what the hell."

Scenario two: You are on your lunch break. You want chocolate. You drive to the little gourmet chocolate shop. You pay two dollars for the dark chocolate, raspberry truffle. Yes, it's a bit pricey for its size, but you remember that what's important is quality, not quantity. The server selects one from the case and places it a little gold box. You sit down at a table in front of the shop. Before you even remove the chocolate from its package you can begin to feel your mouth water in anticipation. You know that you must eat it slowly since there is just one. You gently open the lid. Inside is the truffle, a perfect little orb, deep brown with a ribbon of white chocolate drizzled across the top. You raise it to your nose and inhale its rich, chocolate aroma. You take a small bite and let its smooth filling melt in your mouth. You move it around in your mouth to make it last. The second and last bites are equally deliberate and rapturous. After it is gone, you sit for a moment and let the taste linger on your tongue- Pure Heaven.

Which scenario did you prefer? Which one was the most satisfying?

Now, I don't expect you to make every bite of food a sublime experience, but the more mindfulness you bring to your eating, the easier it will be to be truly satisfied and nourished by your food. Mindfulness is not only important for your "treats" but even more important for your everyday meals. I know that real life is crazy at times. You may have to eat breakfast while driving the kids to school or dinner while catching up on your homework. Mindfulness does not have to be a vow you take and are required to keep. But it is so beneficial that the more you experience it, the reward will reinforce the behavior. So do your best to "just eat" when you eat.

The Scale

The Agony and The Ecstasy

So why am I including the scale in the "mind" section? Because how we think about the scale can make it a useful tool for maintenance or a painful torture device. Let's compare it to a knife. You can use it to make a job easier or you can stab yourself with it. You decide. I know I may seem a bit dramatic, but I have good reason. Remember, for the last 10 years I have weighed people. I'd say I averaged 20 clients per day, 5 days a week. That means that I have witnessed no less than

50,000 reactions to the scale! Most of the time those reactions ranged from mild joy to ecstatic delight, but many, many times the reaction was of intense pain, enough to make *me* cry! Frequently, the scale does not validate our efforts or, for no good reason, shows a gain. It is at these times that I have witnessed the agony that the scale can cause.

One of the most intense reactions that I have witnessed was that of a client who we will call Jane. Jane had been working with me for quite some time to overcome the evening snacking that was slowing her weight loss. Her nemesis was a particular brand of popcorn. Not only was it tasty, but it was also her husband's favorite. This brought emotion into the picture, since they enjoyed sharing it together in the evening. This was the one area that she felt out of control. After many weeks of letting the popcorn sabotage her, she finally got tough. We sat down together before going to the scale. With great pride and a beaming smile, she told me how she had stayed away from the popcorn. I exclaimed how proud I was of her and it was obvious that she was very proud of herself. I felt like I had witnessed her transform into Super Woman! With head held high in excited anticipation, she followed me to the scale. When she stepped onto the scale it actually showed that she had gained a pound! Jane jumped off the scale as if an electric shock filled her body. "No Nika, no!!" she exclaimed with a look of pain and disbelief. The emotion in her voice was as if she had been told tragic news, like the death of a good friend. Her pain shook me also, because I knew how hard she had worked and how proud she was of herself. It was as if the life had drained from her right before my eyes- Superwoman had been hit with Kryptonite-The Scale.

I relate Jane's story because she is normally a level headed, even-tempered woman. She is definitely not someone prone to drama. I sat down with her after she weighed, and it was some time before she regained composure. I tried to console her by commending her hard work and assuring her that, in time, it would result in weight loss. But nothing I could say would remove the betrayal of the scale. Did Jane go back to eating popcorn? Yep. It is what's known as the "What the Hell" syndrome. The feeling that what you're doing makes no difference, so why do it? Sharing popcorn with her husband was more rewarding than the scale, so why change?

The pros and cons of weighing

There can be benefits to using a scale. It is easier to catch incremental weight gain on a scale. You can see immediately if your weight increases. Solely going by how your clothes fit may allow you to gain quite a bit of weight before you notice, depending on how "giving" your clothes are. You may be able to gain up to 10 lbs. before your clothes no longer fit. Most likely if you gain 10 lbs., then you will want to go on yet another diet. That is what we are trying to avoid! By weighing regularly, you can catch your weight gain within 2-3 lbs. and make small adjustments to bring it down, without dieting.

The issue with the scale is that it measures *weight*, not just fat. What makes up your weight? You are comprised of bones, skin, muscles, organs, fat and a whole lot of water! Your bones, organs and skin are likely to remain constant, so that leaves muscle, fat and water. Then there is the content of your stomach and bowels. Did you eat an 8 oz. salad, with 4 oz. of chicken and a 4 oz. apple for lunch? Great choice, but you just ate a pound! Have you eaten that lunch for 3 days and have not had a bowel movement? That's another 3 lbs. sitting in your colon. Did you drink a 16 oz. bottle of water? Good job! There's another pound. Add to all of that, the fact that sodium, hormones, medications, soreness from a work out or other pain causes water retention and you will see why the scale many times does *not* tell the truth. The above example discusses clean eating, drinking water and exercising- all the right things to do, but they can still result in a *weight* gain. Does clean eating, water and exercise cause us to gain *fat*? No way!

Many people have realized that weight doesn't tell the whole story, so they invest in a scale that also reads body fat percentage. They believe this gives them a true understanding of fat loss or gain. Think again. These scales use what's known as bio impedance. A small electrical current is sent throughout your body to measure your body fat. What conducts electricity the best? Water, of course! Hence, the body fat analysis is extremely susceptible to water fluctuation. I have done many experiments on myself and have consistently shown a gain or loss of up to 4% body fat within hours! The analysis was different each time based on not only how much water I drank but also if I had eaten a meal or had a bowel movement. There are also two settings on many high-end machines. Just by changing the setting from "Standard "to "Athletic," It showed that I lost 7 lbs of fat, gained 7 lbs of muscle and dropped my body fat from 20% to 15% in less than a minute. Wow, now that's a diet!

Then there is muscle weight. If you are very active and working out consistently, then a weight gain might be muscle. I say "might" because muscle is not nearly as easy to come by as we would like to think.

If you gain a pound after your morning cardio or even strength training, it is water, not muscle. Remember, muscle fibers are tiny. You can't put a pound on in one workout! Over time though, with consistent strength training, you will gain muscle weight, all the more reason to not get hung up on the number on the scale.

My point to all of this is not to forbid you to ever weigh again. But it is to set you free from the insanity that comes from giving the scale the final say. Why should we let such an unreliable machine exert such control over our minds and lives?

If you choose to use a scale to help you "keep it between the ditches" with your weight management then this is what I recommend: weigh yourself no more than 1 time per week. First thing in the morning, without clothes, on the same day of the week, say Friday. I think Friday is better than Monday. If you're like me, you do most of your dining out on the weekend and usually have a splurge meal or two. Even modest dining out and splurges usually contain more carbs and much more sodium, both of which cause water retention. No matter how minimal I keep my splurges on the weekend, I am invariably up 2 lbs on Monday. And even though I know it will drop off in a couple days, it's still a bummer to see on the scale. Even I have a hard time not getting upset, and this is my profession! So if you also relax a bit on the weekend, don't weigh on Monday, weigh on Friday. If your weight goes up, calmly step away and ask yourself these questions: "Have I *consistently* been eating clean and consciously?" "Have I been getting regular exercise and rest?" "Am I managing my stress appropriately?" If your answer is yes, then it is not fat. It is water weight. Keep calm and carry on. If the answer to any of those is "no" then there is your plan for the week-turn your "no" into "yes." There are a few exceptions. Certain health conditions, medications or serious hormone imbalances can cause weight gain even when you are doing everything right. But from my experience, this is the rare exception. What more commonly happens is that those things are suspected and used as an excuse to not face the truth about our choices. Be honest with yourself; Examine all areas that are in your control, before blaming conditions that are beyond your control. If you do that first and then you suspect medical or hormonal issues to be the culprit in your weight gain, seek medical help. But never use these as a crutch. You can overcome any situation. You are never "destined" to be fat!

KEYS TO CREATING A BALANCED MIND

Silence the negative voices in your head that tell you what you should or shouldn't eat. Recognize that you have the power to choose what's best for you.

Stop labeling yourself as bad, weak and without willpower. Remember other areas in your life where you have shown exceptional strength and apply that strength to your commitment to clean eating.

Bring your brain to the table. Be mindful when you eat. Truly taste your food and be aware of what it is and what it is doing for you.

Step away from the scale! Understand and acknowledge that the scale is nothing more than a tool, and an unreliable one to tell the whole story. Do not give it the power to control your mood or your actions.

Educate yourself regarding the ingredients in your food. Reflect on whether those foods strengthen or weaken your body.

CHAPTER 3
CREATE A STRONG AND BALANCED SPIRIT

Getting to know the true you

W HAT IS THE SPIRIT that I am encouraging you to strengthen and balance? There are a lot of definitions to the word "spirit." The one that fits my usage best is as follows:

Spirit: "the nonphysical part of a person that is the seat of emotions and character; the soul." Synonyms are soul, psyche, inner self, inner being.

When I refer to your spirit, I am discussing the inner you, the real you, your authentic self. Who you are intrinsically, after everything else is stripped away. I am also referring to what I believe is universal and transcendent in each of us- a strong, resilient, and invincible nature. The triumphs of the human spirit are beyond comprehension. When we hear stories of bravery, courage, or survival through unimaginable odds, we are hearing of the strength of the human spirit. Stories such as Ann Frank or Victor Frankl and how they not only endured the Nazi Holocaust, but through it all, believed in the goodness of humanity and a meaning to life. We know of stories such as Oprah Winfrey who rose above poverty, sexual abuse, rape, pregnancy and the death of her infant son at 14 years of age. She became the greatest black philanthropist in American history, using her billionaire status to help others. We could fill volumes with the multitude of present day examples of ordinary people accomplishing extraordinary feats. Their stories exemplify the triumph of the human spirit.

That same spirit is in you. It is in every one of us. Could the same spirit that enabled mere humans to stand strong against the Nazi's enable you to stand strong in the face of chocolate chip cookies? You bet ya! Could that spirit get you out of bed on a cold morning to work out at 5am? Definitely.

Do not underestimate the power of your spirit. Through it you can accomplish great things, and maintaining a healthy weight in our society is a great thing. There is much against us in our quest to listen to our spirit, but the effort yields unimaginable benefits.

A calm and comforted spirit

One aspect of our society that makes it difficult to get in touch with the power of our spirit is our busy lives.

The world is shouting for our attention, but our spirit whispers. It takes a concentrated effort to hear its whispers. There are many ways that we can get in touch with our spirit, but they all require two things, time and silence. A common trait of those that achieve incredible results in life is self-reflection. This self-reflection allows you to evaluate your choices, to decide if they are wise. It allows you to ponder the past, improve the present and plan the future.

Spending time finding out who you are and what you stand for is crucial to making wise choices. Listening to your spirit and drawing strength from it is key to facing challenges successfully. The amazing thing is that you don't have to struggle to find answers to your challenges; You just need to give your spirit the space to speak.

Meditation is a tool used by many to tune into the spirit. Shutting out the noise of the world and spending time being "present" allows you to get to know your inner-self. It is not necessary to have a formal meditation practice, if that doesn't appeal to you, although I encourage you to keep an open mind and explore that option, as the benefits are many. But "meditation" takes many forms. Have you ever sat on the edge of the water, fishing pole in hand, watching the bobber on the surface of the lake? Have you sat on a porch and watched hummingbirds zip back and forth around a feeder? What about lying on the grass and watching the clouds make shapes in the sky? These are examples of meditation. All these activities result in a calm and peaceful frame of mind. The common denominator in these is that your mind is at rest and has a singular focus. This reduces stress and allows the creative mind to emerge. It is in these times that our problems are solved and our path becomes clear.

Another activity that produces peace and clarity is going for a walk. Not a "power walk" where you rush along, perhaps listening to headphones or thinking of how many calories you are burning or all the problems you must deal with when you are done. No, to gain the meditative benefits of a walk, you must truly be present. Feel the ground beneath your feet, the sun on your skin, and the wind in your hair. Hear the sound of the birds in the trees, smell the flowers as you pass by. That is being truly present. You have likely experienced times where a long walk resulted in the answer to a perplexing problem becoming crystal clear. Or perhaps you were in a heated argument and just "walked away" only to realize after your time out, that things were not as bad as they seemed or that you were now able to see the other person's point of view. It is in these times that you are connecting to and nourishing your spirit.

A nourished spirit

How does "nourishing your spirit" help with main-taining your weight? It reduces the tendency to look to food alone for comfort. I say "alone" because I do believe that food can and should be comforting. I do not subscribe to the Spartan "eat to live" mantra. It is the denial that food is a pleasure that inevitably backfires. I believe food is a great sort of pleasure and comfort-and a much needed one. A bowl of steaming soup and crusty bread on a cold winter day is heaven! The trouble begins when food is our only comfort, when our soul cries out for comfort and we stuff our body to drown out its cries. This is when "emotional eating" becomes harmful.

We may be aware that we are prone to emotional eating. After becoming aware of the tendency to turn to food for comfort or stress relief, we may rely on sheer will power to break the habit. Let's say that you had a stressful day at work. You are physically and emotionally exhausted. Perhaps you feel overwhelmed and discouraged as well. "Oh, how nice it would be to dive head first into a package of Oreos!" you think as you drive home from work. As you head for the grocery store, you catch yourself and remember that this is a habit that you want to break, so you get tough with yourself and drive home without the cookies. You are briefly proud of your willpower. Now you have arrived home without cookies but you still carry the stress, exhaustion, and sadness that you had, as well as the added feeling of deprivation because you "can't" have what you want. This perfect storm of emotion now overwhelms willpower, and in desperation for relief you raid the kitchen cabinets. Before you know it, you have eaten a whole box of crackers, the only carbs you could find, since you won't keep "junk" in the house! Now you are stuffed, depressed and ashamed on top of the stressful feelings that you had when you left work. And guess what? You still want the damn Oreos, because the crackers just didn't cut it! Does this scenario sound familiar?

It is one that I have seen all too often. As dieters, we get good at telling ourselves "no." We know that we shouldn't turn to food for comfort. We know in our heads that chocolate won't really improve our job, our love life, or the multitude of other problems we face. But in telling ourselves no and *avoiding* food for comfort, we have left a *void*, an empty place. Our spirit is still crying out for relief, something to take away the pain and give us comfort, security and happiness. If the only way that we know to do that is with food, then we will inevitably turn to food, because the void must be filled.

So what is the solution? Instead of saying "no" to emotional eating, ask "What can I say 'yes' to?" What will bring me relief, comfort and happiness? "

Food appeals to our need for pleasure through the sense of taste. But we have four other senses that can be pleased. Let's look at ways that we can comfort ourselves through the use of our other senses.

We can gain pleasure from our sense of sight. Spending time in beautiful surroundings can give us rest and a feeling of contentment. When we are feeling "stressed out" we need a "time out." Find places near you that are visually appealing. Is there a park or botanical garden by your home or work? When the weather is nice, these are great places to sit and feed the spirit. In the colder weather you may enjoy taking a break in a bookstore that has comfortable arm chairs that allow you to sit back and flip through a favorite magazine. Libraries provide a warm inviting spot to relax as well. Our local library has lots of comfy chairs and a fireplace. There are also study rooms that allow you to sit in silence-such a rare experience these days!

That brings me to another sense, the sense of hearing. Listening to beautiful music is uplifting to the spirit. You can create the mood that you want by choosing the appropriate style of music, something hard and fast to invigorate you or soft and slow to calm you. Conversely, a lack of sound is refreshing at times. Everyone needs a little quiet time. Find a spot that you can be silent. Take a few minutes to "unplug" and enjoy solitude. I am fortunate to have a chapel near my work that I can go to on breaks when the weather is bad and I am craving quiet. It stays open for meditation through the week. If you have never experienced the "sound of silence" you may be uncomfortable at first. Your mind will likely be filled with noisy chatter. But give it time and it will settle down. Focus on your breathing and let your mind rest in quiet for a time. You will be amazed at how refreshed you feel after a few minutes spent in total silence.

We can also appeal to our sense of smell for stress relief. Aromatherapy has been used for centuries to calm or invigorate the spirit. All you need is a drop or two of essential oil in a diffuser to fill your room with a scent that creates the mood that you desire. Use lavender or chamomile for relaxation, citrus or eucalyptus to invigorate. There are so many different essential oils to choose from. Imagine coming home from a stressful day at work and instead of raiding the cabinets, you draw yourself a hot bath and add a few drops of lavender or geranium and soak for a bit. Which do you think you would feel better after, the bath or the cookies?

Speaking of a hot bath brings me to the sense of touch. Warm, sudsy water on your skin, a soft fluffy blanket, a favorite pair of comfy pajamas are all easy ways to find pleasure through feeling. Have you treated yourself to a massage? Even a half-hour session can do wonders to relieve stress.

You see, we have many more senses to appeal to than just our sense of taste. Don't try to "muscle" your way through emotional eating. Instead, ask, "What other ways can I find pleasure that are helpful and not harmful to me?"

When you say "no" to emotional eating make sure you say yes to a healthy alternative. Treat yourself kindly and nourish your spirit when it cries out for comfort instead of trying to silence it with food.

You may think "That sounds wonderful, but I don't have the time for all of those things!" I understand and empathize, but I encourage you to see the importance of it and begin now to take steps to simplify your life. Getting rid of non-essential time drains allows you to create the space to practice self-care. Work toward a simpler life. Stop burning the candle at both ends. Downsize, minimize, delegate and "just say no!" I know it's not easy, but it is crucial to maintaining a healthy weight. Look honestly at your life and ask yourself what activities you can let go of to make more time for you. It may take time to simplify your life, but start now. Your mental, emotional and physical health is at stake-not to mention your waistline!

Another way in which we can nourish our spirit is by avoiding the people or activities that drag us down or "suck the life" out of us. It has been said that we are the sum of our five closest associates. Who do you spend the most time with? What effect do they have on you? When you are with them do you feel inspired and uplifted, or drained and depressed? Do they encourage you to eat healthy and be active or do their comments or example influence you to be apathetic and lazy? It is easy to be influenced by another's negative spirit. We must be on guard and do our best to minimize or eliminate relationships that tear us down. This not only applies to people, but also to our social media and television viewing. Being involved in social media can bring great benefits. I have learned so much through being connected to others in this way. I have been introduced to resources that I would not have found elsewhere. There is much positive information to be found, but there is also much negative. The same questions that I encouraged you to ask for the people in your life I encourage you to ask for your social media as well as your television choices. What we read or listen to is very much "feeding" our spirit. Are you feeding on content that is "nutritious" to your soul? Does it leave you feeling nourished and strong, or drained and weak? There is an overwhelming amount of "junk food" for the brain that we come into contact with every day. The good news is that we can choose not to partake. Make no mistake, you are being fed by everything your eyes and ears take in. Be diligent to protect yourself from those influences that can ruin your mental and spiritual health.

A resilient spirit

Having a resilient spirit is essential for managing your weight for life. Being able to bounce back after difficulties is not always easy. Most people are successful at managing their weight through "calm waters" but fail when they encounter "stormy seas." There will always be circumstances in life that throw us out of balance. Some events that lead to weight regain are a move, job change, new romantic relationship, the sickness or death of a family member, to name a few. At these times it is completely understandable that your weight is not a priority. But even though it may not be priority, it doesn't have to fall by the wayside. We all fall down at times when life overwhelms us. What matters is not that we fall down but that we get back up. No matter what difficulties we face, we can always ask "What *can* I do?" Maybe you are staying with a loved one at the hospital. You may not be able to make your own healthy home cooked meals that you were accustomed to, but you can choose the healthiest item in the cafeteria. Maybe your new job requires more hours from you and you are not able to go to the gym five nights a week like you would prefer. But you can go for a walk on your lunch break. Get the picture? The important thing is that you avoid the trap of thinking, "Let me just get through *this*, then I will have time to focus on my weight." I have seen people put off taking action for years because they fooled themselves with thinking "But next (week, month, year) things will be better. I will focus on eating healthy and exercising then." I hate to be the pessimist here, but how do you *know* that next week or month will be better? It has just as much of a chance to be worse! The point is that you and I cannot foresee the future. All we truly have is this very moment. So yes, hope for a better tomorrow, but take action now!

A humble spirit

Having an honest and humble spirit is also a necessity for maintaining your weight. What does honesty and humility have to do with it? If you are honest with yourself when you need help and have the humility to ask for it, you will not have to suffer alone. You will take action and reach out for help before you regain a significant amount of weight. When I meet with clients that have gained 20 or more pounds back I often ask "What prevented you from asking for help when it was only five or ten pounds?" In nearly every case it was two reasons. First, it was the stubborn declaration of "I know what to do; I should be able to lose it on my own." The second reason is that they were embarrassed to ask for help. Being honest about your need for help and being humble enough to ask for it will enable you to get a hold of your weight when it is manageable and requires only small changes to lose a few pounds. Remember the goal is to never diet again. When you catch your weight gain within a few pounds, it does not require going on another diet. It requires small adjustments, usually just stopping what you were doing to gain the weight: mindless snacking, stress eating, eating out too often, and so on. If you allow yourself to gain a significant amount of weight before you ask for help, no doubt you will feel desperate and miserable and want to go on a diet to lose the weight quickly.

There is no need to get to such a state of desperation. An honest spirit acknowledges that we are imperfect humans. A humble spirit asks for help.

It is difficult for most people to ask for help with their weight. Nearly everyone says "I know what to do" and they believe that this knowing should prevent them from needing to ask for help. But that is not the case. Let's illustrate it in this way: Do you know how to swim? Most likely you answered yes. Then I am sure you would be quite fine swimming alone in your own swimming pool. But what if you found yourself in the middle of a storm- swept ocean? Would you still know how to swim? Sure. You didn't lose the knowledge. Would you call out for help anyway? Of course! Even though you were normally a good swimmer, the conditions and circumstances made it too difficult to go it alone. In this scenario you would be more than happy to accept help.

So how does that example apply to weight management? In my experience people usually do well maintaining their weight until a "storm" of some sort hits-something out of the ordinary that changes their circumstances. This could be a negative event: A sickness or surgery, a death in the family, a job loss or move. It could also be something positive: getting engaged, going back to school, getting a job promotion, taking an extended vacation and so on. What all of these scenarios have in common is a change in conditions and circumstances. There are many events in life that can cause us to lose our focus on maintaining a healthy lifestyle. Even if our life is relatively calm we live in a society that is definitely "storm swept" when it comes to food. Whole books have been written on the sad state of affairs with our food choices today and all the influences against us. So if you currently live in an industrialized nation, you are in the storm as well. The key is to recognize when our personal storm gets too overwhelming and call out for help the first time you feel yourself going under.

Do not feel embarrassed to admit that you are having difficulty making healthy choices. Reach out for help from a trusted friend or family member. Get support from those that helped you to lose the weight. Get involved in a group or community dedicated to healthy living. Whatever you do, take action quickly. Don't allow yourself to be half-drowned by the time you cry out!

KEYS TO CREATING A STRONG AND BALANCED SPIRIT

Recognize that the same spirit that enables humans to show extraordinary strength through hardship resides in you

Nourish your spirit by appealing to all of your senses, not just taste

Reduce or eliminate association with people or media that display a negative spirit and drain your positive energy

Show honesty and humility by asking for help at the first sign of trouble

CHAPTER 4

PLAN B

What if you do gain it back?

MY PURPOSE IN WRITING THIS BOOK is to give you the tools to maintain your weight loss for life. I strongly believe that creating a strong and balanced body, mind, and spirit is possible. If we care for ourselves mentally, emotionally, and physically, our bodies will thrive at their natural, healthy weight. But I also acknowledge that, in spite of our best intentions, life happens. Here's my own example. I had been a weight loss consultant for three years when I met my husband, Larry. We fell madly in love and married within months. Life was magical and filled with lots of dates to wonderful restaurants. He made me feel like a beautiful goddess. So much so, that I hardly noticed my expanding hips and emerging muffin top until I had regained 15 of the 30lbs that I had lost. This happened gradually over a year. Keep in mind that during this year I was a full-time weight loss consultant! So I well know the difficulty in "practicing what you preach." For most of that year I called my weight gain "happy fat." Well, as my first year anniversary approached, I was no longer so happy with my fat. I wanted to fit back into my wedding dress. So I went back "on program" to quickly lose what I had gained. That was several years ago and I have been maintaining within 3-5 lbs since.

My reason for weight regain was a happy one, but for many people it is a negative event that causes significant weight gain. What if you find yourself with enough weight to lose that you want to go on a diet again? Is that so terrible? No, not as long as you learn from it. After all, "There are no failures, only learning opportunities." I am not anti-diet; I am anti-endless diet.

I want you to escape the horrible hamster wheel of continual diet and regain.

That is no way to live. The mental, emotional and physical damage that perpetual dieting does to a person is immense. I want you to break free. But if you are at a weight right now that you cannot be happy maintaining, I empathize. Take action to bring your weight down to a comfortable and realistic weight. But choose your diet wisely. There are many healthy diet programs. Choose one that uses whole, real foods and allows you to lose at a safe and maintainable rate. Going to extremes inevitably backfires. Honor your body by making sure that even though you may be restricted, you are still eating enough wholesome, nutritious food. Honor your mind by refusing to adopt the "diet martyr mentality" by beating yourself up with shoulds and shouldn'ts, good and bad labels. Honor your spirit by choosing a diet that includes food that you enjoy and fits well into your lifestyle.

Do the diet, lose the weight, and then be determined to keep it off for life! Learn from your experiences. Life is too short to be on an endless diet. Think of how fulfilling your future will be when you no longer focus on *shrinking* your waist line, but on *growing* your whole self: Body, Mind and Spirit!

Weight maintenance is an ongoing project. The very word "maintenance" implies continual upkeep, just as is the case when we maintain our home or our vehicle. But living in a clean, well-kept home and driving a reliable car is definitely worth the effort, wouldn't you agree? Do not be discouraged by the fact that you must work to maintain your weight loss. Is there anything worth having that doesn't require hard work and sacrifice? I can think of nothing more worthwhile than doing the work necessary to create an energetic, strong and healthy body. Can you?

Who are you?

Perhaps the most important key to maintaining a healthy weight for life is to create a vision of the person that you truly want to be. Every choice that we make is creating our future self. Every bite we take, drink we swallow, and exercise we do or don't do, is creating either a strong, healthy body or a weak, sick one. Many people gain their weight back because their original reason for losing it was an external one: to look good in a swimsuit or their wedding dress, to feel comfortable during their beach vacation, or to impress friends at their high school reunion. While external goals can definitely help to keep us focused during dieting, they are of little help in maintaining our weight loss for life.

I recall a client who was always focused and successful at losing weight every time that he had an upcoming vacation. He put his mind to it and was incredibly disciplined and lost weight rapidly. Then we wouldn't see him until his next vacation. In between, he would always gain his weight back and then some. But a new, exciting, upcoming vacation gave him the motivation to diet, again. This pattern continued for years, and unfortunately still does.

Does that scenario sound familiar? Yes, America plays it out every summer. Magazines, infomercials, and diet products warn of impending doom-"Summer is almost here! Are you ready? Get that beach body now!" But what if we were motivated by more than those short term, external events? What if our goals were intrinsic, ones that came from within, that aligned with the person that we truly know that we are capable of becoming?

Ask yourself, "Who am I?" and "Who do I want to become?" You are a strong, capable individual, and you can choose to be anyone that you want. The beautiful thing about life is that each new day is the opportunity to begin again. How long will you be willing to live in a fat, tired and sick body? Are you okay with losing weight every summer just to gain it back every Holiday season? Are you willing to play the victim in your life and let yourself sink into the ocean of heart disease, diabetes, and the plethora of other health issues that are plaguing our nation? Or do you want to be a victor, a person that puts your own health as a priority and consistently makes choices that show that you have self-love and self-respect? Will you pass up the donuts because you have a vacation in two weeks, or because you know that all that sugar and refined carbs will do nothing but harm to your body? Will you go to the gym to burn off all the alcohol you drank the night before, or because you want to create a strong, lean, energetic physique? Will you choose water instead of cola because your diet requires you to get 64 ounces or because you know that it will improve not just your weight, bit also your digestion, mental clarity and skin?

Who are you? Are you a victor or a victim? Will you take responsibility for your health and quality of life? You are in the driver's seat. Take the wheel, keep your foot on the gas, and look confidently down the road to your future.

You got this!

BONUS SECTION

10 keys to success for current dieters

THE STRATEGIES FOR SUCCESS in this book are geared toward maintaining weight loss. What if you are not where you want to be weight-wise? Obviously, you must first lose the weight before you can focus on keeping it off. The foundation of creating a strong and balanced body, mind, and spirit as outlined in the preceding are the same for losing weight. The following 10 keys to success for current dieters will distill that knowledge into a guide you can quickly access to help you if you are not yet ready to maintain. If you are starting here, that's great. When finished with this bonus section, go ahead and read the remainder of the book now. It will prepare you for maintenance. Then keep it as a reference after you have lost your weight.

You will find repetition throughout. I am not afraid of repeating myself. We need repetition to truly absorb and apply information. In my work with clients I have seen time and again, just because you told it to them once (or two or ten times) doesn't mean they got it!

Another benefit of repetition is that the information will apply differently at different times in your weight management journey. So I hope you will do as my client and first reader of the book, Sharon, does and keep it on your end table for frequent reference!

KEY #1:
CHOOSE YOUR DIET WISELY

How many diets have you been on? Can you name them? When I've asked clients this, many times the response is "too many to count!" or "You name it, I've tried it!" Why is it that we are seduced by the latest, greatest diet? It astounds me that there is never an end to Women's magazines shouting at us from their stands: "Lose 10 lbs. this week!" "The magic food for rapid weight loss!" "The miracle diet pill recommended by Dr. ..." We jump from diet to diet in hopes of finding the one that will finally work. But what criteria do we use to choose our diet-what our favorite celebrity is doing- What the latest scientific study is touting- Which one that promises the quickest, easiest results?

The sad truth is that most dieters have no criteria for choosing their diet. They have not given careful thought to the standards a diet should meet. Consider how foolish this is. When you decide to embark on a diet, you are agreeing to give yourself over to a prescribed set of rules that will govern one of the most intimate of personal actions-eating.

Eating is the very means of our survival. How lightly we take this critical human need- that of nourishing our very self, of sustaining our own life. The diet we choose will be responsible for rebuilding and repairing the cellular building blocks of our physical being.

Not only is eating a physical act, it is a deeply emotional one. Food brings us great pleasure. It is an integral part of our relationships and culture. The choosing of our diet has far-reaching implications that affect our whole wellbeing.

When we choose to follow a diet that requires us to do such things as drink only liquids or to cut out whole food groups or subsist on concoctions of lemon juice, cayenne pepper and honey, we are causing a whole chain of events. In most cases, these diet extremes cause the body to go into what is known as "starvation mode" where, after the initial quick results, the body slows the metabolism to compensate. This results in our storing fat like a hoarder.

I have known several individuals who have lost drastic amounts of weight on liquid diets, some as much as 10 lbs. per week, only to gain the weight back freakishly fast. One couple I met did only shakes-three meals a day, every day, for over a year, only to regain over 150 lbs just 15 months after they lost it! What must that do to your body? What about your spirit? Think of it-a whole year with no solid food-through all the Holidays, social occasions, events and so on. These liquid dieters are motivated by the insane amount of weight loss and pride themselves on their willpower. Dieters though are human, and humans as all other creatures, seek pleasure and avoid pain. Some hold out longer than others, but such extreme diets never work for sustainable results.

What must a person do to succeed on such a diet?

They must, in effect, cut their eating habits off from their true self. Through desperation and sheer force of will they detach themselves from their food. This is the "eat to live don't live to eat" mentality that personally makes me crazy. This mentality preaches that food is fuel, no more. They behave as if we are simply automobiles with a gas tank to be filled. Not so! Food is a great pleasure and pleasure is a primordial motivation in life. Denying the pleasure factor of food will always end in disaster.

Eating extremely low calories will also backfire. So how then should we choose our diet?

Choose a diet that uses real whole food as its primary foundation. I am not opposed to using some high quality, all natural shakes or bars as long as they are a *supplement* to, not a *substitute* for, real whole food- vegetables, fruits, whole grains, legumes, lean proteins and such.

You should have plenty of foods to choose from. Avoid diets that have every meal specifically planned for you. While you may be seduced by the ease of not having to think for yourself when it comes to meal planning, this will backfire. If, for instance, on day three of your "21-day diet plan," dinner is tilapia and broccoli and you hate fish, what happens when your husband orders pizza for himself and the kids? You will be much more tempted to break your diet when facing the fish then if you had planned a tasty recipe of your own from an extensive list of choices.

Variety not only keeps you from being bored or

tempted, but it can also help weight loss in another way. Different foods provide different nutrients. For instance, oranges offer large doses of vitamin C, bananas abound in potassium, while avocados are rich in heart healthy monounsaturated fats. By eating a mixture of real foods you are covering your nutritional bases.

If our bodies do not get all the nutrients they need they are more prone to fat storage. Fat is a protection for the body, like money in the bank. When we are in need, we are less likely to "spend." So mix it up. Getting variety in your diet will physically help the metabolism, but will also keep your taste buds happy. Why is that so important?

Few things get under my skin quicker than encountering someone with what I call the "Diet Martyr" mentality. Diet Martyrs proclaim " I hate it, but I'm eating it!" They pride themselves on being miserable while dieting. They believe there is virtue in eating foods that don't taste good to them because they are "healthy" or "on the diet." Let me be clear. If your diet does not offer enough foods that you enjoy, you are on the wrong diet.

Many people down play this. They ask "What is the harm in making yourself eat something that you know is good for you? After all, isn't that being a disciplined dieter?" You could look at it that way, and for a brief period, muscling your way through your diet can result in weight loss, but my years of experience with dieters has given me the "big picture" view. There is always a backlash to disconnecting to our true self. The stress caused by forcing yourself to eat something that tastes unpleasant is an actual stressor. Stress causes the hormone Cortisol to rise and our digestion to slow. This results in our not fully assimilating the nutrients in the so called "healthy food" that we are forcing down!

There is a multitude of nutrient-rich foods to choose from. Don't buy into the thinking that you have to eat the latest highly-touted "super food" to lose weight. Now, I will admit that some food is an acquired taste, so if it is slightly unpleasant but you believe it is nutritious, there may be some merit in trying it a few times to see if you can acquire a taste for it. But if you truly hate it, please don't eat it. Choose something else. There is no virtue in crucifying yourself for the religion of nutrition.

KEY #2:
HAVE A CLEAR VISION OF YOUR "WHY?"

Why are you on this diet? What is your desired outcome? When I ask clients these questions, nine times out of ten the reply with something like "to be healthy." Now, that's exciting! Or not. "To be healthy" will not propel you through the hard times. That vague notion will mean nothing when your husband brings home pizza after you have worked a ten-hour day and have nothing prepared. It will not prevent you from diving head first into the Ben and Jerrys after that fight with your boss. "To be healthy" is shallow and weak. It is the opposite of compelling.

Your reason for dieting, your "vision" must compel you, propel you, forward. It must light you on fire and fill you with excited anticipation that is more real and tantalizing than any temptation or challenge you encounter.

Here are some compelling "whys":

- To play with my grandchild without pain in my knees

- To vacation with my family and have the stamina and energy to enjoy it.

- To get the job promotion I desire by presenting a professional appearance

- To feel confident and present the "real me" as I begin dating again
- To set an example for my children to prevent them from developing diabetes
- To lead an energetic, active retirement
- To have a better chance at a healthy pregnancy
- To be a role model for my family.

Do you see the difference? All of the above reasons involve a tangible, happy outcome. You see positive things in your future. Then the work of the diet, while still work, is now exciting because day by day you are creating your inspiring future. Choice by choice, your vision is becoming reality. It is the difference between building your dream house, or just being contract labor, hammering the nails.

Both scenarios involve hammering nails, but building your dream house fills you with excitement for the work. Working as a laborer only is mundane, unsatisfying, and the first chance to quit you'll take!

Notice that none of the reasons above were "to avoid"

- to avoid buying bigger clothes
- to avoid being the "fat mom"
- to avoid heart disease
- to avoid diabetes

But what's wrong with that? Aren't those worthy goals? Maybe, but the answer is in the question- the "avoid" goals leave a "*void*." They all tell you what you are *not* going to be. Okay, so you are not the fat, diabetic mom in a plus-sized dress, but who *are* you?

Feel the void, the nothingness that is left? Not too compelling is it? Your reasons for change must be tangible, positive and passion filled. Find your "why" and hold tight. Eat, sleep and breathe it. Taste it. Savor it. When you find it hard to stick to your diet, I promise you that is because you are losing hold of your "why" or you never had a properly formed one to begin with.

What if you can't find a compelling reason? Then I'm going to ask you to do some soul searching.

Do you really want or need to lose weight? I have seen clients tormenting themselves repeatedly over losing that last five or ten pounds. I help them break out of the purgatory by asking them this- "How will your life improve by being five pounds lighter?" Most have no answer but have held onto the goal for the simple reason that they had that number of their goal weight stuck in their head for so long that stubborn pride prevented them from releasing it.

If your goal weight will provide no real benefit to you except bragging rights that you achieved a certain weight, let it go. Move forward and live your life; it is not worth prolonging a diet, an unnatural state of living, any longer than necessary.

KEY #3:
LOSE THE GUILT

Dieters are often burdened with guilt over their food choices. This is another facet of "Diet Martyr" mentality. When you choose to eat something not on your diet, avoid saying you "blew it" were "bad" or that you "sinned" or "cheated." Food choices are not illegal or immoral, so unless you stole that candy bar or killed someone for it, drop the drama. It's food. You chose to eat it. That choice was not conducive to weight loss. That's it. Learn from it and let it go.

I know losing the guilt regarding food is easier said than done. You may have been shamed as a child for what you ate. Your friends and family may think they are your personal "diet police" nagging you with the judgmental "Is that on your diet?" Even delicious desserts are often labeled "sinful" or "decadent."

Which brings me to the paradox of labeling food as bad. Let's face it, we all have that little side of us that wants to be "bad," to be "risqué," to break the rules. Most of us will avoid acting out in immoral or illegal ways, but what better outlet to be naughty then indulging in a "sinful" chocolate brownie? Am I right?

Labeling our food choices as cheating actual increases our desire for them! At one time, my husband and I were dieting together. We were "on program." As we were driving by our favorite frozen custard stand, he turned to me with a mischievous grin and whispered " Oooh, do you want to be *bad*?"

Knowing frozen custard was definitely not on our program, I replied nonchalantly "It's not bad, it's just not on program." His demeanor changed as if I threw cold water on him. My refusal to view it as cheating took all the fun out of it. He drove away.

See food choices for what they are. Don't give them unnecessary power or allure. Get over the guilt (and the thrill) of so called "cheating."

KEY #4:
HAVE REALISTIC EXPECTATIONS

Another pitfall of dieting is believing the hype about quick weight loss. It never ceases to amaze me (and upset me) that people continue to fall for the incredulous claims made for diet programs or products. Many of these claims are out-right lies, such as the promise that a new diet pill will lead to rapid weight loss without diet and exercise; if that happens, you will be losing mostly water weight and will gain it back quickly when you get rehydrated.

As a weight management coach, I recommend some natural herb and vitamin supplements as an aid to weight loss. Be clear though, that supplements will NOT work on their own. I emphasized to my clients that these were supplements to, not substitutes for, clean eating and exercise. They provide concentrated nutrients. Herbs and vitamins in many cases have centuries of documented health benefits. By infusing our bodies with nutrients, we get a boost that helps with weight loss.

Let me illustrate. There are fuel additives that help your vehicle run better. You add them to your gas tank. What if you added the bottle of fuel additive along with a handful of dirt? What if you drove your car and never got an oil change? How about if you let it sit in the elements without driving it? How well would it run? The fuel additive will not take the place of quality gasoline and proper vehicle maintenance. There are no magic pills. Listen closely. None. Nada. Get over it. Haven't we been gullible long enough to learn to see through the claims?

Also to be avoided is expectations of a certain amount of weight loss per week. While claiming "up to 7 lbs. per week" may not technically be a lie, it is a deception. Why is it not a lie? Notice, It does not say that you WILL lose 7lbs a week; It says "up to." Oh, that little phrase, "up to." It is nonchalantly hanging out on all the weight loss claims, yet it is virtually invisible. No one reads it, no one hears it. Why? Because, whether we want to admit it or not, we usually believe what we want to believe. We want to lose 7 lbs this week and every week, so we silence our voice of reason. You know, that nagging voice that says "If it sounds too good to be true..."

So let's examine what "up to 7 lbs., (or 5 or 3) per week is actually saying. It means that somewhere, some time, someone achieved a 7 lb. loss in one week on this diet. It is not promising that you will. It doesn't even guarantee that said dieter lost 7lbs every week or that they didn't gain 8 lbs. back the next week. It's like purchasing a lottery ticket. There may have been "up to 50 billion dollars" in giveaways, but you'd be a fool to believe that you are guaranteed the same.

While following a nutritionally sound diet, you can expect to lose weight, but you cannot know exactly how much or in what time frame. Our bodies are miraculously complex creations. So many factors determine how you lose weight throughout the course of the diet. I have seen firsthand that it is not just diet and exercise that affect the scale. Other factors that determine our results are our mental state; how well we are handling stress; our pain level, the health conditions, disorders, diseases we have; the medications we take; how well we are sleeping; how frequent our bowel movements are; how much water we retain, and so forth. Because of the multitude of variables involved, the only thing we can reasonably expect is "forward progress."

Barring any serious cases of the above factors, you can expect to lose weight on a good diet, but it will likely be much slower than you expect.

I know that you do not want to hear this, but trust me. In over a decade of weighing clients over 50,000 times on several different diet plans, I'm an expert on this statistic. The majority of diligent, consistent dieters average about 1-2 lbs. per week. Keep in mind that is average, meaning that one week they might lose 3 lbs, the next they might lose one. I tend to go on and on about this because of the sheer agony I have witnessed with the scale. Enough of the insanity! There is no way to know with certainty how much you will lose. Go buy a lottery ticket if you need a dose of fantasy turned to disappointment. Stop playing this drama out every morning when your feet hit the unforgiving metal of the bathroom scale.

Which brings me to the 5th Key to success on a diet-Don't let the scale have the last word.

KEY #5:
DON'T GIVE THE SCALE THE LAST WORD

In case it isn't abundantly clear by now, I have a pretty dysfunctional relationship with the scale. It would be accurate to say I pretty much loathe it. Our relationship hasn't always been sour. In the beginning of my personal dieting saga at 18 yrs. old, I truly believed the scale was my friend, there to help keep me on the straight and narrow. Why the bitterness between us now? Because I came to see that Sister Scale is a back-stabbing, cold and heartless B@#%!

Am I right?

Think about it. How many times has she done *you* wrong? How many times have you worked your butt off- stuck to your diet religiously, resisted temptations like a saint, and exercised with discipline and rigor, only to be rewarded with no loss, or even worse, a gain! "Back stabbing" is right, or more like a knife through the heart. I've witnessed the agony on client's faces week after week, as well as experiencing it myself. "Whyyyyy???" We cry out. Here's why.

The scale does not just weigh fat. Your weight is also comprised of water, blood, bones, skin, muscles and organs. Add to that, the content of your stomach and bowel. Of course, bones, skin, and organs stay relatively consistent throughout our adult life, but water and bowel content vary throughout the day and day to day. Due to these variables, it is sheer futility to weigh yourself more than once a day. In my opinion, even that is too much. Limit weighing to once or twice per week, if you must.

What do I mean, "If you must?" After all, you may wonder how you will know if you have lost or gained weight. Here's how, by opening your eyes and using your brain. You are an intelligent person and can see and feel for yourself. Tune into your body. Can you feel yourself getting smaller, tighter, leaner? How are your clothes fitting? How do you feel? If you will truly connect with your body, you will know if you are making progress.

You will eventually lose weight on the scale if you are losing fat. The exception would be if you are strength training with enough intensity to build muscle. In that case, your muscle gain may be proportionate to or even exceed your loss. This will cause the scale to stay the same or even show a gain. If you are honest and connected to your body, you will know if it is fat or muscle. Here is a clue-muscle doesn't jiggle. Fat is jiggly, soft and voluminous; muscle is firm, hard and tight. Muscle has definition; fat spills over. Don't deceive yourself by thinking that your daily walks are building muscle when the scale goes up. Are your pants getting loose or tight? Muscle, while weighing more, is smaller. So if the scale goes up and the pants are looser it could be muscle gain. Women in particular have to work at it hardcore to expect to gain even a pound of muscle. If you are not training intensely enough to build muscle but you are eating clean then the scale will eventually reflect that, but not every time you step on it. So back away from the frenemy and weigh rarely, if at all.

For many women, weighing has become such a part of our life, it is almost a rite of Womanhood. Not weighing seems a sacrilege and can result in anxiety and a sense of loss. I experienced such feelings when I started to wean myself from daily weighing. I missed it. I felt nervous that I might just go crazy and lose all control without its daily censure or approval. It took some time to release those feelings and break away. I still step on a scale from time to time when curiosity gets the best of me. I don't believe it is necessary to completely abstain from weighing, though that would be okay. Those that refuse to weigh, though are sometimes in great fear of the scale and don't trust their reaction to it. I don't want you to fear the scale. I want you to see it for what it is- a tool, no more, no less, and a pretty ineffective one as well. It is not an indicator of your self-worth, simply of how much physical space you take up on the planet.

As of this writing, I am still employed for a weight loss company and I weigh people for a living. It is my least favorite aspect of my job. But I do it, because we have yet to arrive in the utopian world that I dream of- one in which we have freed ourselves from the scales bondage. Occasionally a client refuses to weigh or to be told how much they weigh. This makes no sense when one has joined a weight loss program that uses a scale. I'm not asking you to buck the system. I am just encouraging you to view your weigh-ins in perspective, taking into account the variables that we discussed above. Simply quit giving the scale power over your attitudes and actions. Stop looking to it for validation of your worthiness.

Spend time getting to know who you are, what you stand for, and what is important to you. Do you want to create an attractive, comfortable body to the best of your ability? Then commit to caring for yourself through proper nourishment and activity. The scale is just a number. Get to know your body and respect and love it for getting you this far in life.

KEY #6:
STOP STUFFING YOUR EMOTIONS

"I'm an emotional eater." I can't tell you how many clients have confided this to me. The confession is usually brought forth through much effort and accompanied by a blush of shame. It is reminiscent of an AA meeting, "Hello, my name is Suzy and I'm an emotional eater." My reaction to their confession usually shocks them- "Of course you are; so am I." What? A weight loss consultant should be above turning to food for comfort, right?

Wrong.

Why wouldn't we turn to food for comfort? Food is the second greatest pleasure known to man...without the strings attached. Kind of like a "friend with benefits." So what benefits does the pleasure of food give us? Oh, I could fill pages with the answer. Food makes us happy, can warm us, or refresh us. It can give us soft and soothing when we are sad or hard and crunchy when we are mad. It can bring back memories of childhood fun, thrilling vacations or romantic anniversaries. Sharing a meal with friends and family is a meaningful tradition in all cultures.

It is a real sore spot for me that the emotional aspect of eating is vilified among much of the fitness and nutrition community. The mantra of "food is fuel" seems virtuous enough on the surface, but let's look deeper. Yes, food is fuel in that it is used to power us. We need to choose foods that nourish and "fuel" us throughout the day. I even used the gas tank analogy previously, explaining that we shouldn't put "dirt in the tank" and expect high performance.

But the problem lies in viewing food as fuel only. We are not just cars with gas tanks. We are complex, emotional beings. We have taste buds for a reason. Denying the pleasure factor of eating will invariably back fire.

The problem is not that we feel emotional about food or that we look to food for comfort. The problem lies in using food to avoid our emotions or "stuff" them down, so we don't have to deal with them. Let me illustrate.

Here is a fact that you may find surprising about me. I have dark chocolate and red wine every night, almost without exception. I have one serving. I look forward to this nightly indulgence. It has become a pleasant ritual for me. After supper, I pour my Merlot into its long stem glass. I buy a type of dark chocolate that comes individually wrapped in black and gold foil. I relax onto the couch in my silky PJs and favorite blanket.

I take small bites of chocolate and a sip of wine simultaneously, allowing them to mingle together on my tongue. Wine and chocolate meld together like perfectly-paired lovers. It is an exquisite dance of flavors. What a lovely way to wind down the evening! On particularly stressful days I look forward to this ritual all the more, because I know it is "me time" to slow down and treat myself. Do I sound emotional about my wine and chocolate?

Absolutely! This in an example of beneficial emotional eating. Not only does my splurge of choice have the heart-healthy benefits of antioxidants, flavonoids, resveratrol and such, but even more importantly, they make my figurative heart happy as well.

Now let's take another scenario-one of harmful emotional eating.

Imagine that I have come home from work angry and stressed. I grab the bottle of wine and whole package of chocolate and eat and drink several servings in quick succession as I fumed over the day's events in my head. I'm not tasting the wine and chocolate; I am using them to numb my emotions, to stuff them down. I'm looking to get drunk and sugar crash to avoid how I am feeling; I would've been just as well with cheap beer and M&Ms! Do you see the difference? Do you *feel* the difference?

The key to not stuffing our emotions with food is to learn other ways to find comfort and release from stress. Food delights the sense of taste, but we have four other senses. Look for ways to satisfy the senses of sight, smell, sound and touch. Stress relief is anything that makes you happy. What makes you feel safe? What makes you laugh? What smells good to you? Who can you talk to? What can you read that will up build you? There is a multitude of ways to find comfort other than food; It just takes thinking "outside the box." The box of cookies that is!

KEY #7:
LEARN FROM IT AND LET IT GO

"There are no failures, only learning opportunities"

One of the ways that dieters self-sabotage their weight loss efforts is by having a perfectionistic, "all or nothing" mentality. The moment they have a slip up; they feel that they have "blown it." They then mentally beat themselves up for being too weak or lacking the willpower to succeed. Discouraged, they give up, throw in the towel, and slide back into their old ways.

This results in them gaining even more weight, until the pain of it causes them to try again. If they bring the old perfectionist thinking with them into the new diet attempt, they are doomed to fail once again.

How can we stop this insane loop of self-sabotage?

By recognizing that we cannot fail, as long as we learn from each slip up. By suspending self-condemnation and examining what went wrong, we can learn. Having learned, we can adjust our actions in the future. Learning from our mistakes allows us to "let it go" and not be overwhelmed with guilt or disappointment.

"Success is going form failure to failure without loss of enthusiasm" said Winston Churchill. Those words were spoken to troops regarding war-time battles. Surely they can be applied to "battles" with weight loss!

Let's look at some common scenarios that lead to diet failures and see what we can learn from them to succeed in the future.

One of the most common diet fails is having a moment of weakness when tempting non-diet foods are present. There are several reasons for this. First let's look at the physical aspect. Many times we are tempted because we are simply hungry and experiencing low blood sugar.

Our brains run off of blood sugar, so when it is low our thinking ability is impaired.

Blood sugar lows are the result of not eating the right foods at the right times in the right amounts. So let's examine how this could play out.

Scenario #1
The Candy Dish

Imagine that it is 3pm and suddenly the office candy bowl has irresistible appeal. It calls your name, tempting you to come closer. You don't understand its overwhelming allure, since it has been there all week and you've not been tempted in the least. But today is different. You reach your hand into the bowl and indulge in the forbidden fruit. No one is around, and since you feel that you have already "blown it" you have a couple more handfuls. Once the sugar orgy is over, you are left feeling ashamed and wonder how you could've been so weak.

Have I described this scenario with candid accuracy? That is because I have lived it more times than I care to recall. After giving into temptation it is easy to conclude that we will never be able to conquer or sugar habit, that we just don't have the willpower necessary. But let's see what we can learn from this example.

If we carefully analyze our actions, we may determine that we did not eat enough lunch so we were extra hungry. We may realize that fatigue contributed to our desire for a sugar "fix." Hungry and tired do not strong will power make. After reflection, we can choose to eat a more sustaining lunch tomorrow, as well as getting to bed earlier at night.

Diet Fail Cause: hunger and fatigue

Diet Fail Cure: Eat a sustaining lunch; get adequate rest.

Scenario#2
Pizza Night

It's Friday night. You've had a long, hard, work week and arrive home worn out and starving. When you open the front door, the aroma of "hot and cheesy" envelops you. At the kitchen table your family is freely indulging in their usual Friday night pizza- fest. You try to summon your strength and resolutely walk past them to the refrigerator. Inside, the only diet-friendly food is frozen chicken and whole vegetables. You know it will take time to defrost and cook the chicken as well as to cut up the salad. Besides, chicken salad feels like punishment compared to pizza. "Oh screw it! I'll get back on my diet tomorrow!" You promise as you dive head first into the pizza. You eat several pieces in quick succession before getting a grip. Now you are left wondering what came over you and begin the self-beating for lack of will power.

So what did come over you? Again, fatigue and hunger were prime factors, but this time the deciding factor was lack of preparation.

You got too hungry because you waited too long to eat. Lunch was at noon and now after 7pm your blood sugar has dropped too low. If you had brought a small snack to have before arriving home, you would've been able to wait until you prepared your meal.

Another lack of preparation was not having something equally quick and tasty as the pizza on hand. By preparing food ahead of time, perhaps a crock pot recipe or casserole that could just be reheated in a few minutes, you would've had a tasty alternative to the pizza.

Forethought and planning go a long way. Start planning for recurring pitfalls such as Friday Pizza Nights. Unless you secretly really just want pizza, then own up to that! It is always your choice; no need for excuses.

Diet Fail Cause: Too hungry, not prepared with quick and satisfying options

Diet Fail Cure: Bring a snack to work. Prepare a reheatable meal ahead of time that is appetizing or plan to count pizza night as a spurge meal to enjoy with family.

Scenario #3
Girls night out

So, you're a social butterfly, the life of the party. It's just not a "girl's night out" without you! You stick to your diet all week, but when the weekend comes, your efforts are derailed by cocktail hour. I can't tell you how many times I've seen this scenario played out. Many times it is much easier for us to give up our favorite foods than to give up alcohol. I get it, and that doesn't necessarily have to qualify you for a 12 step program either! When I was dieting, my nemesis was that beautiful glass of red wine while dining out. When sharing a nice meal with my husband, I feel that wine "elevates" the meal, making it all the more special. I paid too much for that fancy meal to insult it with a boring glass of water! I soon realized though, that wine was slowing my weight loss and sabotaging my efforts. What did I do? I got tough and decided that I wanted to lose weight more than I wanted wine, so I quit ordering it. To ease the pain I ordered sparkling water with a lime wedge and requested it in a nice glass. That was all I needed. I realized that it was more about the experience than the actual alcohol content for me.

What's wrong with a little alcohol while dieting? Even if you choose low calorie, low carb options, the issue is with the alcohol itself. When alcohol enters our body, it has VIP status. All efforts go toward metabolizing it. Fat burning takes a back seat. You basically disrupt the fat burning process until the alcohol is metabolized.

Any food you consume with the alcohol is not burned well either. The problem is compounded because alcohol lowers inhibitions, often then leading to poor food choices. After a couple of glasses of wine, that dessert menu is looking mighty sexy!

Back to girl's night out. A lot of psychological elements are at play here. The desire for fun, to not be a "bummer" and not stand out as different is a real challenge. Peer pressure can be real as your girlfriends urge to have "just one drink!" So how can we avoid that pressure?

First ask yourself this: Who are these girls? Are they your true friends? If so, then they would undoubtedly have your best interests at heart and readily understand your abstinence. Wouldn't you support your true friend's choices? If they do not support you, wouldn't it be safe to conclude that they are not your true friends after all?

Now, chew on this: Are you going to let the opinion of someone who is not really your friend, who does not have your best interests at heart, determine your diet success or failure? Stand up for yourself, girlfriend, and stop living for everyone else. Make up your mind and stand firm! Never be embarrassed to do what you need to accomplish your goals.

You can ease the situation by being the DD as well. But what if it isn't peer pressure? What if *you* feel like you are missing out? Remind yourself that this is only temporary. What are you really missing out on when you keep failing your diet? If you think about it, you are missing out on your best life. Always remember the big picture and grasp that your choices are taking you closer or further away from your desired future.

Diet Fail Cause:
Social drinking temptation and pressure

Diet Success Cure: Acknowledge the impact that drinking is having on your efforts. Recognize that true friends support you; false friends don't matter. Order sparkling water with lime. Be the designated driver. Visualize yourself at your goal weight, having a drink then.

KEY #8:
DO YOUR PRESENT BEST

> *Do what you can, with what you have, where you are*

-Theodore Roosevelt

"I can't..." How many times have dieters given up with these words? "I can't join a gym." "I can't afford healthy groceries." I can't work out because of my knees." "I can't cook separate meals for myself and my family. "I can't find time to work out." I can't, I can't I can't!

Many times, this is simply a lack of prioritizing our health and wellbeing. We all have 24 hrs. in a day and our money is being spent on what is important to us. That being said, there are some legitimate "can'ts" as well.

Let's examine " I can't join a gym." This may be true for a number of reasons. Perhaps the budget truly doesn't allow it at this time or there are no gyms (or decent ones) in your small town. Maybe you have a domineering spouse who is opposed. (I will save my "Leave his ass!" speech for another time.) I have actually been in all three of those scenarios. What did I do? I found alternatives to the gym. I walked outside. I bought an inexpensive pair of adjustable dumbbells and a plastic step for cardio. I lost 20lbs with that equipment alone.

What about "I can't exercise because of pain in my knees" or other painful conditions? Exercise what doesn't hurt. Do upper body strength training. Swim if you have access to a pool. Do low impact Pilates or Yoga.

There are endless possibilities for exercise.

What about having to cook two meals, one for your family and one for your diet? Most of the time moms are able to find healthy diet-compliant recipes that their family likes as well. I understand, though, that some families are just not willing to give up their unhealthy favorites. When the family demands chicken nuggets and mac and cheese, what's Mom to do? Perhaps get some help with the cooking. Is there an older child in the family that might pitch in and help cook? If there are no other options besides cooking two meals, then cook two meals. You are worth it! Chicken nuggets and mac and cheese will bring more harm to you in the long run than making the effort to cook something better for yourself. Be smart and plan ahead. Make foods that are easy and make several servings that you can reheat. Success requires effort. Do what it takes to fill your needs as well as your families. Besides, if they see you eating healthy, over time you will likely influence them. The day you hear "Ooh Mom, can I have some of *yours*?" You will know that your hard work and example paid off.

Why did I entitle this section "do your *present* best?"

Because so often people put off taking action until they think conditions will be right. "Next Monday" becomes next week, next month, next year. "When the kids start school" becomes "When the kids are grown" "When I finish college" becomes "When I get a better job" becomes "When I retire" Do you see the depressing theme here? The point is, life never slows down or smooths out completely. Our future slips through our fingers while we wait for a better time. The time is *now*. Do what you can at this time and in this place, with whatever means you have.

" If you can't fly then run. If you can't run, then walk. If you can't walk then crawl, but keep moving forward"- Martin Luther King Jr

Get in the habit of asking "What *can* I do?" Then do it!

KEY #9:
FOLLOW DIRECTIONS

"If all else fails, follow directions." How many times have I heard "This diet isn't working" when the truth of the matter is that it was the *dieter* who wasn't working! Diets work in a variety of ways. There are many ways to manipulate calories or macronutrients to prompt fat burn. Each diet must be followed the way it was designed to work correctly. Diet plans are like puzzles; you must have all the pieces and have them arranged correctly. The puzzle picture will not turn out right if you are missing pieces, add in pieces from a different puzzle, or arrange them incorrectly. So during a diet, if you miss foods, add in foods that are not part of the diet, or don't arrange your meals properly, you will get frustrating results. Find a diet you can stick with, using the guidelines discussed in Key #1, and follow it as written. If after giving it your best effort, you decide it is not a good fit for you, then you can choose not to follow it. But is it fair to blame the diet if you have not followed it correctly? Poor adherence equals poor performance. Diets do work, when we do the work.

I know that diets are difficult to stick with. This is because a diet forces the dieter to eat unnaturally. It is my wish for you to never diet again, but I understand the desire to lose weight quickly. I recognize that most people are reluctant to stop dieting, hence my inclusion of these 10 keys to success. So view the diet as a temporary "necessary evil." Be strict and get done with it! Don't half-heartedly attempt a diet for months or years. You have a life to live, and the closer you adhere to your diet, the quicker you can go about learning how to reverse the "dieter mentality" and live like a normal human being with a healthy relationship with food. That is the purpose of this book.

KEY #10:
SEE PAST THE DIET

A diet should have a definite beginning and end. We should approach it the same as other challenging endeavors. For instance, let's compare it to training for a marathon. During your training you know that you must live differently than non-competitors because you have a challenging goal with a specific end-date. You know that to complete the marathon, you must train, even when you don't feel like it. You have chosen to live abnormally to get a desired result.

We can also compare a diet to getting your college degree. You study and attend classes even when you don't feel like it because you have a specific graduation date in mind. You live differently than non-college students. You may stay home and study, when you'd rather be out with friends. That is known as dedication. Dedication breeds success. Think of areas such as these that you have shown dedication to achieve a desired result. Apply that past dedication to your present diet efforts. Do the work and show the resolve. Repeated diet attempts slow your metabolism and damage your wellbeing on all levels- physically, mentally and emotionally. Life is too short to be on a perpetual diet. Do what it takes to attain your goal weight and get off the endless diet merry-go round.

Okay, Now what? Most dieters rarely think of "life after

diet." This is like only planning for a beautiful wedding with no effort made to create a beautiful marriage. What is your plan for maintaining your weight loss for life? What healthy habits must you continue to keep the weight off? What skills will you need? How will you learn balance when the rules of the diet and the rewards of the scale are no longer there? The word "maintenance" implies consistent, regular work, just as in maintaining a home or vehicle. With continued practice, maintaining your weight will become natural, and will no longer occupy such a large part of your consciousness. You will then be able to truly enjoy your life, free from diets forever. You can create true strength and balance of body mind and spirit, resulting in a joyful relationship to your food and your life.

I hope these tips help you to succeed in your weight loss journey. Managing our weight requires consistent, conscious awareness of our choices, but after some time it becomes second nature. I encourage you to go back to the beginning of this book to learn how to gain the physical, mental, and emotional strength and balance to maintain your weight loss for life. Never give up. You are worth it!

Congratulations on taking the time to become a loser and a keeper! I would be honored to assist you in your weight management journey. Visit me at

nikaford.com

for more education, empowerment, and inspiration!

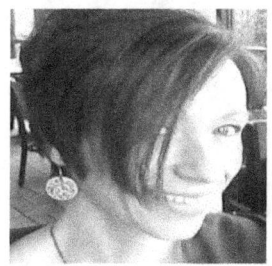

ABOUT THE AUTHOR

Nika Ford is a Transformation Coach and Author with more than ten years' experience with weight loss consulting. She is committed to empowering and inspiring lasting change.